THIS BOOK

BELONGS TO

....

....

Thank you for Purchasing my book and taking the time to read it from front to back. I am always grateful when a reader chooses my work and I hope you enjoyed it!

With the vast selection available online, I am touched that you chose to be purchasing my work and take valuable time out of your life to read it. My hope is that you feel you made the right decision.

I very much would like to know what you thought of the book. Please take the time to write an honest and informative review on Amazon.com. Your experience and opinions will be of great benefit to me and those readers looking to make an informed choice.

With much thanks.

@COPYRIGHT 2024

Table of Contents

1

WILL I EVER GET PREGNANT?

For a smart and intelligent woman, reaching all the milestones of success, including graduating from college, getting a higher degree, and landing a stable and successful career, is a goal. A little later, you want to find love with a partner you want to start a family with. Even if you might have suspected that getting pregnant might take a while, nothing could have prepared you for experiencing infertility.

It is difficult to accept failing at something that should come naturally. As each month goes by without getting pregnant, the panic starts to take over. Questions that you want the answers to, but don't want to ask, are:

- Will I ever get pregnant?
- Am I too old?
- Will I have to do IVF?
- Are my eggs still good?
- If I do get pregnant, will the baby be healthy?
- What should I do?

- Who should I ask?
- How do I know that what the doctors are telling me is true?

Being smart, you probably think you should know all the answers, but sometimes being smart is what works against you. Having focused on a career, thoughts of waiting too long or making the wrong decisions about pursuing a successful career haunt you. You may be asking yourself, "Why can't I figure it out?" Additionally, you may be going back through your life and trying to determine where you made a wrong decision.

Perhaps you found your partner later in life after securing an advanced degree, getting a career going, and feeling confident and stable. Previously, you might have thought that "happily ever after" was for other people, but as things seemed to line up, you thought there might be hope for you too. When you met that special person and got married or decided that you were committed, everything changed around starting a family. Something kicked in, and it seemed like your whole life would collapse or be meaningless if it is childless. Maybe you think that if you can't get pregnant and have a baby, your spouse or partner might leave or love you less; maybe you will love yourself less.

Everywhere you look, you get the same statistics – if you are over thirty-five years old, and even worse, if you are forty, you have a less than 4 percent chance of getting pregnant naturally. The odds of having a baby with a genetic disease increases and the chance that a pregnancy will have many more health risks is even higher. This means that you don't have the time to go the "normal" route. You missed that fertility window of opportunity where one night of unprotected sex will get you pregnant.

Looking for answers online, reading books and blogs, and searching for reasons why you are not getting pregnant – like your age and your weight – can make you feel helpless and hopeless. You try to solve these problems on your own and feel like your life is upside-down as you struggle to achieve the ideal diet, exercise, and lifestyle that can help you get pregnant. After going into chat rooms, you find yourself changing your diet radically to meet the optimal fertility health. This still may not be enough, as being a bit older has a ticking biological clock. Having waited already while you pursued other life goals, you cannot put having a baby on hold; in fact, you needed to be pregnant ten years ago, according to doctors.

Without undergoing invasive medical procedures and taking poisonous chemicals, the doctors are not even sure they can help you get pregnant. This can make you feel like you missed the boat, so to speak, showed up on the wrong day when the party is over.

It seems like everyone else is able to get pregnant easily and that can make you feel happy for them and sad for yourself. As someone who is smart and who has figured out so many things in life, wondering why you haven't been able to get this right can be the most difficult experience you ever have to deal with.

It's so easy to feel ashamed of where you are. As much as you can put on a brave face, the feelings that you did something wrong, took a wrong step, or somehow missed your chance of having a baby follow you. You may ask yourself, "What is wrong with me?" However, the terrifying response is that there is no true answer. Even if there is something "wrong" and you know how to fix it, it could be too late.

At this late stage, you get the same answer everywhere – your eggs are probably too old, and your only real chance is to get IVF. Even then, there is no guarantee. You may have already tried a couple of fertility treatments at a fertility clinic, where you woke up every morning to get your blood taken, injected yourself with hormones, and hid what you and your spouse were doing from family and friends in order to avoid painful conversations, not revealing how much pain you felt. Sometimes you even held back from sharing that pain and suffering with your husband.

The whole point of a family is to make the relationship with your husband closer and have a child from the both of you, one you can love and raise together. A child would be the evidence of your love for each other; you never wanted the journey to leave you feeling like you are alone. Even this, you can't share.

What is frustrating is that you have been doing everything "perfectly." This is the high standard that you hold for yourself, but this time, it's not working, and maybe it will never work. Every child's birthday party and every baby shower invitation are reminders that you are not experiencing that joy of motherhood, and it brings that terrifying fear that you're missing out on one of life's greatest joys.

If you could wake up one morning, pee on that stick, and see the plus sign to signify that you are pregnant, you would have your husband go to the drugstore and buy a few different pregnancy tests to check, double check, and triple check that you are not dreaming. You dream of the first sonograms, the heartbeat, the excitement, and the anticipation of finding out if the baby is a boy or girl, as well as wondering who it will look like and getting to tell your family and friends that you are expecting a baby.

You want to experience the incredible, warm feelings of gratitude that wash over you, knowing that there is a beautiful baby who will come into your life. You envision finding out that you are pregnant with a healthy baby and that you will hold this happy and healthy baby in your arms nine months from now. A little being will come into your life to love and take care of, and you will watch them learn to sit up, turn over, crawl, walk, talk, and give you tiny little hugs and kisses. You dream of reading bedtime stories and playing in the park. You get to see the wonder of the world through a child's eyes. Wouldn't that be splendid?

For now, life is on hold. Everything revolves around trying to get pregnant and looking for answers as to why it's not happening. This is extremely taxing on your relationships, especially with your partner or husband. The romance is gone, and sex is about timing for reproduction. You wake up in the middle of the night with your heart racing and a lump in your throat; it's like you are being choked, the life is being suffocated out of you. You don't want to answer any more questions like, "When are you and your husband going to have kids? Are you thinking about starting a family soon?" You just want to go crawl under a rock. You just don't feel like seeing friends or family because it takes too much energy to pretend that everything is fine when they give you that funny look.

Looking at the financial costs that add up from doctor visits and what rules your insurance has about fertility treatments makes it feel like everywhere you turn, it is getting more and more difficult to move forward. How can you put a price on having a baby? The money makes it harder to know what the right thing to do is.

Maybe you have been hiding all this from your employer by making excuses as to why you have to leave early or come in late. There may be the prospect of surgery or needing a donor egg. How far will this go before you break? Those options cost more than money; they cost your health as well.

You dream of coming home with a little smiling baby in your arms, knowing that you will experience motherhood and that you and your husband will be parents and love that little baby, watching as he or she grows up and feeling pride over getting to be part of your child's life. You want to love and teach your baby, watch them grow and learn, take first steps, say first words, make friends, and give you hugs and kisses. You want to share your life experiences of growing up, going to the beach, camping, and going to school. You dream of giving your baby all the love you have, the things you wished for, and getting to throw a first birthday party and go to Mommy and me classes. The best part of all of this is that a child is a creation from you and your husband and a deeper connection to share your love.

I understand that you are at a stage of your fertility journey where you are experiencing the pain of not getting pregnant. You may even feel a loss of a future that has not yet been determined and are careful not to let yourself hope too much so you won't be disappointed. You are not alone in these feelings, and it is completely normal to feel what you are feeling, but also know that in the next chapters I will share what you can do, so your future will have your baby in your arms, smiling up at you.

2

DISCOVERING WHAT WAS WORKING

As an alternative and Chinese medicine practitioner with over eighteen years' experience, I administered somewhere in the order of forty-five thousand acupuncture and herbal treatments to patients and trained over seven hundred acupuncture practitioners, including some MDs. I came to specialize in fertility as women are 90 percent of my patient population and they tend to be between the ages of thirty and forty-five. Most often, the subject of having a baby is why they seek acupuncture and natural healing. In my experience, women will tend to be more open to alternative medicine and will look for ways to heal outside of mainstream medicine when it is failing them. Helping women who struggle with infertility heal underlying health conditions so they can get pregnant naturally became my area of expertise.

Each woman who shared with her family, friends, and mommy groups of how I helped her have a baby after struggling spreads the knowledge that there is hope for getting pregnant and natural alternatives through acupuncture, herbs, and energy healing. In Chinese medicine, every aspect of health is considered, even family health history.

Many of my patients ask me how I ended up becoming a Chinese medicine practitioner and specializing in fertility. I realize that Chinese medicine is not the first place that people look to solve general health problems. In fact, most people will seek everything else and be up to their eyeballs with specialists and Western medicine until it repeatedly fails them miserably. Eventually, frustration and disillusionment drive people to seek something else by stepping out of the proverbial box to search for an alternative.

No one grows up wanting to be a Chinese medicine practitioner. In fact, I didn't know anything about it. Like many aspects of my upbringing, my attention and education were pointed in a direction toward fitting in, and that meant the white, Anglo-Saxon aesthetic. There was not much about acupuncture and Chinese medicine that would reach the ears of this little girl, although I do have some memory of seeing an acupuncture needle in my father's lower leg, though I'm not sure where that memory came from.

Chinese medicine and acupuncture are a mysterious kind of knowledge. I owe a debt of gratitude to James Reston, whose shared experience with acupuncture became a catalyst for acupuncture and Chinese medicine to be recognized in the United States. Acupuncture and Chinese medicine entered the homes of everyday America in 1971. As a *New York Times* journalist covering President Nixon's visit to China, Reston ended up having an emergency appendix operation and reported being treated with acupuncture and moxibustion in the hospital for pain. Mr. Reston was conscious during the surgery and had a speedy recovery.

Prior to that recounting of his experience, acupuncture and Chinese medicine were obscure and a mystery in the United States. Chinese medicine was only available in Asian communities and through family traditions. Practitioners of martial arts had techniques for bone setting and trauma healing that is part of Chinese medicine and further developed because of the frequency of injuries due to the nature of the sport. The herbal recipes would be handed down by masters and were part of the *dojo*, or martial arts school/club.

Martial arts is considered, or can be considered, a branch in Chinese medicine, as it recognizes the flow of life energy, *qi*, through channels and movements. In martial arts, there is the drawing of universal energy and breathing, allowing a connection to the earth and the heavens. Tai qi and qigong are the same forms used in martial arts only done slowly with the intension to move energy through the body and connect with nature and universal energy. Injuries are treated not just as a sprain or bruise but with the idea that the body must heal itself and restore the free flow of energy.

The events in my life came together and made sense to me as to why I chose this path.

Growing up with the values of working hard, getting good grades, and fitting in also meant not being "too Chinese." My father, an immigrant from China, became a Western medicine doctor in the 1950s. He achieved the American dream and believed that was the highest status achievement you could have, aside from being a Supreme Court judge. My mother, also in medicine, was a nurse, so you could say I grew up on Western medicine.

Inhaling the sweet smell of medical journals lying on the bedside table in my parents' bedroom, I looked at grotesque pictures of diseases, sniffing each page to see if the pictures' smells revealed some secret information, an example of a child's wonder and curiosity.

Sitting on my father's lap, I would draw pictures of the digestive system and get approval for knowing where the organs were. On my father's days off, he would go on rounds in the hospital and my brother and I got to go too, visiting patients and greeting the nurses and doctors on call or waiting in the doctors' lounge.

Early experiences in childhood can create very strong impressions that later carry over to the choices we make about what we want to be when we grow up. That was the case for me; when I was seven years old, I got appendicitis and spent an entire month in the hospital. The abdominal pain I had seemed to not "fit" appendicitis, so the doctors had trouble diagnosing it. I was poked and prodded, X-rayed, put on IV fluid only, drank chalky drinks, and there was no diagnosis. Eventually, I was operated on for exploratory surgery and my swollen appendix, the size of a small cucumber, was removed. After being a seven-year-old stuck in a hospital and experimented on, you could say that my trust in people wearing white coats was broken and that the adults in charge lost my confidence. My appendix experience had a profound influence on the direction I took in the future.

Throughout my teens, I worked in my father's office and I spent two summers as a volunteer in the hospital. My dad talked with the hospital administrator and arranged for my brother and me to have hands-on experience. I spent that time in the basement in central supply (next to the morgue) and my brother in the emergency room, but the following year, I spent the summer in the OR and recovery room, glimpsing surgeries, cleaning operating rooms, and watching and comforting patients as they groaned in pain and emerged from anesthesia. Though I was being groomed to go into medicine, I was actually learning about what was missing in medicine.

Something I notice in so many women looking for answers for their fertility struggles is that they find that there is something lacking – missing information. There is someone sitting with a stethoscope, a white coat, plenty of plaques, and a lot of letters after their name, and you think they will know more than you, but I found, just as I did when I was seven, that doctors are people and Western medicine does not have all the answers and searching for alternatives will help you get pregnant.

While I was interested in medicine because of being exposed to it at home through my parents, my personal experience in the hospital left me with feelings of emptiness and dread. As much as the doctors were doing their job to find out what was wrong, they did not see me as a whole person – the little girl, scared and isolated from her family, friends, and school. I was getting care, but what was missing was the personal connection and compassion. This is not to say that doctors do not care; in fact, some doctor mask their empathy by being "professional." However, as a child, it came across that they did not care about "me." This experience left an impression on me that I did not want to become a doctor.

So instead of going into medicine, it seemed like working in "business" would be the right direction to take. Working and making your own money was a value that was instilled in me early on in life. If I wanted something, I would have to "earn money" to buy it. This was my father's way of teaching me the "value" of the dollar. He worked his way through college and medical school, so he felt that it was important that there was an "earning" lesson in everything. Personally, I wanted to work in an office with air conditioning and that was "business" versus being a laborer. I worked three jobs and went to school at night for college. I got a lot of experience in various industries from working for a designer making samples and cutting fabric, to corporate travel, to then running a US division for an Italian leather goods company, but when the economy faltered, working in the fashion luxury goods business was no longer viable; the company decided to close their office. I then worked for a domestic accessories company. It was miserable. By the time I finished my degree in business, I was "over" corporate culture.

After pursuing a career in the business world, I found it empty and questioned if what I was doing was making a difference, thinking, "What is it that people need? What is it that I need?" The response was massage therapy. I had looked at becoming a massage therapist once, many years before, because I felt how healing it was. It just hadn't made sense for me until then. I started massage therapy school at the Swedish Institute, and during that first module of shiatsu and Eastern Foundations in medicine, it became clear that I would continue on to study Chinese medicine. It was then that Chinese medicine made so much sense that I could help people become whole with their health and awaken their innate healing power. What I ignored, and even rejected culturally and spiritually, was the path I chose when I accepted being a healer.

Why fertility? It is no surprise that women seek out healing and alternatives to heal themselves. I had a baby in my last year of acupuncture school and was an "older" mom. I studied a lot about women's health and Chinese medicine and was fortunately immersed in this process of cultivating health for myself. I understood how precious it was to have a healthy baby and thought about how it might not have happened and the great loss it would have been. From the side of having the baby, I know how special it is, and I would not want anyone who desires to be a parent to miss out.

There is another driving force as to why I wanted to help women, and it is because women are the underdogs. Women are not well attended in medicine. The old ideas of women being hysterical because they have uteruses still seem to echo the way women are similarly placed on birth control and antidepressants. I see how Western medicine is molded to continue to perpetuate and subjugate women around their greatest power and that is to reproduce.

The moment we step into a doctor's office, there is a power differential. In an instant, we assume that the doctors know more about our bodies than we do; they are the experts. There is truth that they do have expertise in what they do, but it is important to recognize that medicine as practiced has been based on bias. Women's biology is not the same as men's biology, so if medicine is based on a male health model, women will always be off and not conform to a textbook example.

The medical training and science backed research has inherent, internalized biases, so when you do step into that medical office environment, it will feel like someone taking over your biology with authority and making you feel like you are unworthy or incomplete. This is what happens all the time with fertility and cancer treatments. The "problem" seems to conclude that women are weak, and this opinion is formed from a male perspective; this is an invisible force that is all around us and we, as women, act upon it as if it was true.

Western medicine was developed from a male point of view and its culture is dominated by white male privilege. We, as a culture, default to assumptions that men are superior and women are less-than. This is where we can end up, handing our power over to a system that is dysfunctional, and this is why it does not feel good to be treated in Western hospitals. Somehow we know it is not right, but without awareness that there are other possibilities, we feel we have no choice.

Perhaps because I am an Asian American woman, I observe the subtle ways that I am treated here in the United States; aside from my gender, there are a lot of assumptions made about my demeanor, such as being quiet, deferential, and exotic. These assumptions are known as orientalism. Being treated a little differently raised my awareness even more about how medicine is not impervious to cultural bias, and that is what drives me to open other possibilities for women who want to have a baby. It takes courage for a woman to step outside of that paradigm of not being "allowed" to think of her own body, as her own property, and deciding that you are in charge.

I believe women need to be in charge of their own reproduction – their body, their choice. There are thousands of years of medical knowledge of women's health well-documented in Chinese medicine, and it would be irresponsible to ignore the experiential data. Taking advantage of the best of both Western and Eastern medicine makes sense. Our tendency to look at choice as either/or can seem like we have to swap one for the other, but the power is being able to blend and integrate.

Early on in my practice of Chinese medicine, a woman who sought treatment for infertility taught me how difficult the journey was and the suffering in silence that she could not openly share. She did not talk much about the doctor appointments or her numbers or even her anxiety and how she was suffering with the trying process. What I observed is that the more stress and fear present, the more a woman will stay quiet and cautious when talking about infertility. This has often been the case with something as painful as infertility. Silence can be a great teacher and a woman showing up in deep "pain" from wanting to get pregnant and have a baby is her vulnerability that she shares. I can share with you the story of my patient, Emilia, and how her courage and action helped her overcome the pain of doubt and despair to succeed in getting pregnant.

One of my patients, Emilia, related her story to me when she came for treatments. Emilia shivered when she laid on the table. Though terrified of needles, she was doing whatever she could to make that last intrauterine insemination cycle count. She was working another job on the weekends so that she would have some money for acupuncture, massage, and chiropractic visits. The single room office was warm and cozy and located on eleventh and Broadway, with a chair in the hall to wait. As the practitioner, I stayed in the room, writing notes and being careful to stay quiet while she rested during the sessions. The jagged scar on her lower right abdomen was a reminder of a lost fallopian tube from an ectopic pregnancy. The wave of sleepiness and warmth spread through her body as the effects of the needles took effect. She would soon be forty – the dreaded "age" that fertility clinics sometimes refuse service, but all that seemed to melt away as she drifted in and out of sleepy relaxation. I could feel Emilia's anguish, yet she was doing everything in her power to increase her chances of getting pregnant. She was courageous in the face of disappointment and fear.

I am so grateful that she came to me and trusted that I would be able to help her with acupuncture and Chinese medicine, and I did. I was a witness and held space for her to heal. This is a miraculous collaboration between the patient and practitioner, a synergic meeting of the mind and heart for both.

This great healing energy that we all have inspires me to help women who struggle with fertility to heal underlying health issues, so they can get pregnant and hold their happy and healthy baby in their arms. For me, those birth announcements and pictures of first birthdays, first tooth, Halloween costumes, pony rides, first day at school, the missing front teeth, and holiday cards, are where I get to see these babies become little people who are a mix of their parents. There is immense gratitude when I can help bring forth another life into the world by going up against the odds and the patriarchy that not only exists in our culture, but definitely also in medicine and profoundly with women's health and reproduction.

I love being able to help women become mothers because it is something so much more than biology, and it frees women from the hopelessness that Western medicine often prescribes. There is process of getting out of this model of health that is hopelessness and fear, and it means we will be taking a journey with some steps. They are not necessarily linear, but I have found that there are critical topics that need some attention and will addressed in the following chapters. These steps helped so many women overcome their infertility and are a guide for you to use and overcome your infertility challenges. Each woman who shared with her family, friends, and mommy groups of how I helped her to have a baby after struggling, spreads the knowledge that there is hope for getting pregnant and for natural alternatives through acupuncture, herbs, and energy healing.

In this book, I will share many of these patients' stories with you, whose names and some details have been changed for privacy purposes.

3

THE MAP IS NOT THE TERRITORY

know that when we are in a hurry we focus on the destination or what the secret ingredient is to a recipe, so in this chapter, I will teach you how to use this book.

It takes a lot of courage to do this, so I want to acknowledge this quality of exploration in you. Just taking that step means you are already doing something different, and that is what you need to keep in mind. Consider that you are like other women, but not the same, so as we move through the book and steps, there will be parts that will seem more relevant to you; bear in mind that you have some blind spots or beliefs that may trigger you. If there is something that you disagree with or feel strongly about, observe it and be curious.

This book is for women who are ready to step outside of their comfort zone and try something new and different. Writing this book is to bridge the gap of all that scientific and medical knowledge you have most likely consumed and to help make sense of how it relates or does not relate to your fertility journey.

There are more steps to getting pregnant and having a happy and healthy baby than what the medical community addresses or will even acknowledge. That creates a big gap for women who are struggling to make sense of where they fit in. Often, women are not a perfect fit for the programs and procedures. In my practice, how I work with women in my program originally was going to be called fertility boot camp, but I found that women were already in their own kind "boot camp," getting intimidated and pressured to conform to a certain standard. So instead, I called my program "The Fertility Goddess" to embody that we all hold the God and Goddess power within us.

This book is a roadmap to help you get from struggling with infertility to taking steps to getting pregnant. We will be connecting some dots, so to speak.

One of my favorite quotes is "the map is not the territory." Most of what we "know" is processed through our filters of reality, and if we acknowledge that we have these filters, we can also try changing our filter to see a more "complete picture of the territory" and try another route.

Doctors and fertility clinics tend to look at their patients from one lens and viewpoint. The metaphor that is often used is the "single tool approach," and that is a hammer, and everything needs to be molded into a nail so that they can use that one tool. I liken this approach to what I do, as my approach is more of a Swiss army knife with lots of tools that are adaptive and can be useful beyond fertility.

You can always go back to what you were doing before, but now you will be able to gain some more knowledge and information. In this book, we will be unpacking some myths about fertility and why they are detrimental to you getting pregnant. You are sure to see that some of these may relate to you.

We will also be looking at the big picture of health and what leads to reproductive health; this is often "touched" on and also often ignored.

At this point in your reproductivity journey, you may have been told that you have a particular issue for why you can't get pregnant, but I know that you would not be reading this if you thought that was completely true.

We will discuss topics such as the biological clock and fertility doctors in Chapter 5, priorities in Chapter 6, creating a fertility plan in Chapters 6 and 7, health and fertility testing in Chapter 7, removing energy blocks in Chapter 8, perfection sabotage and charting in Chapter 9, healing relationships in Chapter 10, feng shui in Chapter 11, and the power you have in Chapter 12. You might decide that you "know some of this information already," but even though you may have heard this information before, the information presented in this process will be a new experience.

It is important to not skip ahead.

This is something that I notice with smart people – they can get a concept quickly but pulling all those things together to make them work is where the challenge lies. If you ever had to put some IKEA furniture together, you will notice that every piece is accounted for, and if you don't read the instructions carefully, you end up having to take the whole piece of furniture apart. Even when reading the instructions, you can sometimes go on autopilot and do something else and then have difficulty and get lost. The steps in the book are not a hard-and-fast order, but for those who are doing some of the processes already, do not skip or ignore the steps, because you may feel like the information is disjointed. In some of the steps, you might have to reread, as there is novelty and even some resistance. That is also part of the process and is completely normal.

The first few steps are like backing out of a dead end and getting to a road that leads you to familiar settings so you can navigate to your destination. Moving through the book, some steps will seem strange, or you may even question why they are important, and that is okay. New concepts will bring up resistance and skepticism. You don't have to like them; you just need to give them a chance by working with them.

There are exercises that go with each step so that you can implement them immediately and start to get the health benefits.

This means that you don't have to read the book first and then put it into practice; the book can be used as a guide as you are carrying out each step.

I liken this to going to the gym and exercising; you can understand the concept of exercising – the goal of losing weight and getting fit – but unless you stick with it, you will not gain enough of the experience and physical evidence that it works. The greatest lesson for people who train or study is sticking with it, and that comes from experience. Give yourself a chance to experience the process.

We will go through exercises to help shift your energy because when experiencing infertility, staying in the energy of hope and faith are what will give you that nudge to keep moving forward.

You will hear real stories from my practice of women and couples who struggled with infertility, and how they overcame their struggles. There are also women that have had a first child that then experienced an inability to have a second child, known as secondary infertility.

We can't leave out the partner or spouse who is part of this fertility journey; the toll that infertility takes on couples is tremendous, and you will learn how to create a deeper connection as well.

You will also learn about obstacles that have been invisible to you because they seem innocuous, but once you become aware of them, you can fix them.

Additionally, you will be shown how to create a plan that keeps you from going crazy through your fertility journey so that you can continue to move forward and get pregnant.

Let us begin, and in case you are wondering when to start, you already have, so let's continue! In the next chapter, we will get clear on our bearings and why you are on this journey to become a mother. It may seem like it is obvious, but I have found that getting some clarity helps to sort out all the overwhelming feelings that can show up at this stage of trying to get pregnant.

4

THE BIG WHY

If you were sitting in my office, the first question that I would ask you is, "Why do you want to have a baby?" This might be kind of a shocking and strange question to ask, but it is important question to answer and understand before going forward. It may seem like a big, "of course I want a baby," but the question is not whether or not you want a baby, it is about why now. Sometimes we struggle with wanting something so badly that we don't even remember why we wanted it in the first place. When it doesn't happen, we can feel like a little piece of us is dying.

After struggling and being met with failures, searching for answers, and getting lots of misinformation, we pick up a lot of garbage and scary thoughts. If this was a radio wave, this would be static interfering with the journey.

Imagine you are going to the grocery store to pick up eggs. It is a simple thing to do – go to the store, find the eggs, and go to the checkout counter. However, when you get to the dairy section, there are tons of types of eggs – grade A, jumbo, brown, free-range, omega eggs, organic, non-GMO, organic brown, local eggs, store brand eggs, eggs in cartons, eggs in clear plastic, and eggs on sale.

There are so many options to consider. Which is better? Now, you might have heard about GMOs and how they are bad and that maybe organic is best, but they are three times as expensive, and they look the same, and then why are eggs on sale? Are they going to go bad? Which eggs do you buy?

What just happened? A lot of information intruded on the simple activity of buying eggs, and it suddenly became a bigger decision-making process that can lead you down the path of distraction and uncertainty.

Why did you want to get eggs in the first place? How about to make an omelet? With wanting to have a baby, there is a lot of distraction and information that comes up about how to get pregnant, and that interferes with that desire; it doesn't mean that you don't want it, it just makes the *why* of it gets muddied.

The moment you decide to have a baby, a flood of information about how to get pregnant and what you need to do when having a baby comes in and perhaps puts the brakes on your momentum. Maybe you feel like your dreams are being squashed just a bit when the searches come up with age viability, health, egg quality, and a bunch of diseases that make you go down a rabbit hole, searching for answers for something you don't even have. With every possible block that shows up and makes you discouraged, you can lose sight of your *why*; this is why knowing your *why* is so important for your success.

When I ask, "Why do you want to have a baby?" there is often a pause, and then the woman may search for the "right" answer like, "I'm getting older and it's time to have kids," or "my siblings all have children," or "we just bought a house." But I know that is not their true why. Often it is in the form of a feeling and a drive.

The next questions I ask is, "What will it do for you to be a mom?" This is when the big why shows up – the bigger piece of a strong desire that is connected to your being. To bring a life into the world, to love this baby, and raise it to be a wonderful person. The why is the miracle of life – something that is greater than a biological function.

The why is your desire. In Chinese, there is something called *zhi*. Its closest translation is "will," "determination," or "purpose." The character 志 represents grass above; it is the symbol of the heart/mind, pushing the plant above the ground, to come into existence. This closely relates to many sayings, such as "where there is a will, there is a way." Your why will activate your will; this involves connecting your heart/mind to that desire that is within and to push through the ground and bring forth new life into the sunshine.

I remember attending the graduation ceremony for medical school at Columbia. It was a warm day in June, set in a garden area, and my daughter was one year old. As the presenter of the diplomas spoke and gave out the certificates, he talked about how the families that were seated had also gone through the process, supporting the graduates financially and emotionally, and this was also part of their celebration too. They too experience the years of studies, sleep deprivation, rotations, and passing the boards to finally get the degree. The most heart-opening moment was that with each diploma, there was a copy of the graduate's essay that they wrote when applying to medical school. It was what inspired them to become a doctor. I love this example, because along the way to committing to something, we get caught up in the *doing* that we forget the pure reason *why* we are doing it.

Is becoming a parent something you always wanted?

On a scale of one to ten, where are you with your desire to have a baby? Anything below an eight means you probably would not be reading this book; ten is a burning desire.

I have found that, with women who always envisioned that they would have children, there is something that makes it inevitable, a type of unwavering commitment to continue in the face of adversity. There is something that I have also noticed, and that is that little girls who have strollers and dollies and pretend to be moms have something innate inside of them – a desire to nurture something. I also know that is not a guarantee that those little girls will grow up to have children, but it is the energy of love, care, empathy, and parenting.

Why do you want to have a baby? Take a moment and feel this question. This is something that will help you shed all that static. Answering the *why* clears out all that extra stuff. For some women, they can feel it is part of their purpose, that their life would be empty if they were to miss out. Somehow they know that it is the most important thing for them right now.

Do you have a clear picture? This is a moment where you can connect with that image and the feelings that are a part of it. As an exercise, I recommend creating for yourself a vision board where you add the images and symbols of what it will mean for you to become a mom. There is no right way to do it; it can have pictures of toys, or puppies, birds' nests, a school, a park, whatever represents your desire to be a mom and is relevant for you. This is a way to express what you are feeling right now – your why – and how you see yourself in the future already having that beautiful baby. Think of it as a place holder and an inspiration to keep you moving forward.

Later we will do more exercises. I put this one here so I wouldn't forget to remind you how important your *why* is and that images are stronger than words. You know what will move you and make you smile.

Your *why* is the constant on your journey and should not be confused with *how* it will happen. You may have a lot of questions about *how* this will work. Bringing a new life into being is no small feat, and according to scientists, the probability of you being born as you are is one in a 400 trillion. It is amazing that there are so many humans on the planet! When I heard this statistic, in a weird way, it did make me pause and think about how the conditions have to be just right for those cells to come together to form that human being – the human being you will birth into the world. It also made me think about how special everyone is and that there are more than hormones, eggs, and sperm at play.

There is much we don't understand about the universe, but we can still witness it unfolding. This why I like quantum physics, because there is the concept that there is more than one possibility existing at any given moment – that we can exist in many timelines and that all things are possible. What was also observed in quantum mechanics is called the "double slit experiment," and when the experiment was "observed" by scientists, the particles and photons behaved differently than when they were not "observed." This meant that by looking at something, we influence it on an atomic level.

So, why do I bring this up? What we focus on tends to grow, so it is important to keep a soft and steady gaze and an eye on the prize, so to speak.

Your *why* will help you step out of conformity and the status quo and defy statistics, which I consider a type of evil because they tend to provide information that has led many women to make choices about their fertility based on fear. Fear is one the strongest emotions we have because it triggers survival; this means we will see things in terms of life and death and black and white. When your nervous system is switched to this mode, your brain will not allow any new information to penetrate, and your ability to make an informed choice is not readily available.

The more we want something and focus on it, there is an aspect of trying to control the outcome. In doing so, we get stuck in the *how* something has to happen. This is placing conditions on what has to happen versus the conditions that will bring about success. When we place conditions on what we want, we inadvertently push away what it is that we desire because we do not keep our *why*.

Have you heard the saying "how you do anything is how you do everything"? With fertility, this is where it is easy to lose your way. The static that we pick up on the journey to having a baby, like "I'm too old" or "I'm not healthy," is one of those things that blocks us; it also creates a lot of stress that makes getting pregnant all the more difficult. The focus gets into how we have to do this fertility thing, and when we also buy into why it is not working, we further find ourselves in despair. As you are aware, this also creates of a lot of stress. The more we have obstacles that jump into our path, the more we take on stress. I say "take it on" because we choose to focus our attention on what we think is important and it causes a lot of unnecessary stress.

Doubt creeps in, and you might entertain thoughts of giving up. When you embark on a big journey, like having a baby, a lot can show up to stop you. I will go over some of this in subsequent chapters.

So again, on a scale of one to ten, where are you in your desire to have a baby? Why might you give up? When I ask this question, it is not to squash any dreams. On the contrary, it is a hard look back on how you might approach what it is that you want. It's important to look at what point someone would give up.

Is there anything that you can see that might stand in your way? Do you feel that having a baby is not in your control? Is it up to the doctors to determine whether you can have a baby or not?

Candace was a woman who wanted to have a baby. She was married for some time, and she and her husband never really thought they would have difficulty with conception; there was an ease and care with their relationship. Other than with her parents and in-laws, urgency was not there. She was confident that she would get pregnant, but it just was not happening, and as she turned forty-one, the statistics were starting to appear against her favor. She sought fertility specialists, and they were discouraging. She did several cycles of in vitro fertilization (IVF) treatment that failed.

She and her husband were going to spend a few months in New York City, and they would do their last IVF cycle at a clinic. Candace came for treatments, and she had a determination and optimism that create great energy. That energy was there until she was into her IVF cycle. The doctor was trying to "manage her expectations," indicating that her age was a problem and that it might not happen, especially since it was her last IVF cycle. The physician perhaps thought he was being helpful in some way, but most likely to buffer his clinic statistics, he told her that "maybe she was not meant to have a baby."

As you could imagine, this hurtful comment was the opposite of inspiring hope or possibility. In these moments, when I hear this crap, it is infuriating to me. How dare someone ever say that. It is a spiritual *wrong*. As a mom, I felt like I was being stabbed in the heart and could not imagine what Candace must have felt, but it was not good. I also know that if this were a man, no doctor would ever suggest that maybe they were not meant to procreate. I am certain that the remark was not intended to be hurtful or discouraging. Doctors are doing the best that they can with the methods and tools that they have learned to use.

Candace was a strong woman and did not allow this insensitive remark to drag her down. We recognized that this had nothing to do with her and her ability to get pregnant; it was about the doctor's confidence in his own ability as a fertility specialist, perhaps placing his own value on whether his patient could get pregnant. Her desire to have a baby was very clear and transcended any hurtful words. She was clear about why she wanted a baby, and she and her husband were without doubt that they were doing the right thing. The outcome was that nine months later, she delivered a beautiful baby girl.

I observe a lot of misinformation, discouragement, and even shame when women want to have a child. It is tragic that family members or well-meaning friends say things that are hurtful and can keep these women from continuing on.

The most important part of this journey is that you don't forget your *why*. Your *why* is what will help you continue on your journey to have a baby – no matter what.

FERTILITY WORKBOOK EXERCISE

Write yourself a letter of why you want to have a baby. Answer the following questions:

- Why is it important to you now?
- How will it feel?
- What will it do for you to be a mom?
- What do you envision when this little baby is in your arms?

This letter/essay is where you create a safe place to share with yourself in this moment in time. What this letter will be is a reminder of your why and how big this desire is; you can read it anytime, like a trusted friend with your secret. By putting it in words and on paper, you have created a possibility that now exists in a physical form.

There may be some doubts that come up or voices of why you can't or shouldn't become pregnant, and one voice in particular may have to do with age. The topic of age and getting pregnant can be discouraging, so my suggestion when writing is call it something else, such as "my beach balloon," and take the charge out of it. In the next chapter, we will be unpacking the topic of age and how not to let that control your destiny.

5

AM I TOO OLD?

Many women wonder, "Am I too old?" Why do you think that? Chances are, you have been reading some statistics on women, fertility, and age. The medical profession is not kind to women and uses words like "advanced maternal age" or "geriatric pregnancy age"! These are labels for women over thirty-five years old and speaks to the underlying ageism and misogyny of the Western mind-set that influences medicine. Unfortunately, the attitude toward women and reproduction resembles that of livestock.

Biological and chronological clocks are not the same. One size does not fit all. There are many women over thirty-five who have conceived naturally and delivered healthy babies. There are also women forty-plus, mid-forties, and late forties who also got pregnant and delivered healthy babies, some even in their fifties. The problem is that we just don't have the data. Fertility statistics come from women who are seeking help because they are struggling with getting pregnant, but that is not all the women! You have to be careful not to throw yourself into a category that is not true.

You are not broken. We have a model of health and medicine that is known as a "broken and fix" model. If you are seeking help for a "problem," the assumption is that you are broken. When you want to have a baby and you have been trying, it is easy to jump to the conclusion that there must be something "broken," and you might feel like you are broken, but the one factor that keeps getting your attention is that you are over thirty-five years old, so that must be it. However, you can't change your chronological age and that is what can lead you to desperation – looking for a solution for your "age." You will then be focused on how to solve the age problem and not look at your whole health.

Because the model of medicine is segmented and specialized, you can end up going further and further into data and statistics until you look at subatomic particles. Can you ignore the birthdate on your driver's license? This is going to be something that you will need to ignore.

Fertility is big business, and when you start searching and inquiring, you will be offered a protocol. This is purely based on your age, without having any tests that will be offered to you based on your age. Fear that you may be too old will push you in the direction of getting IVF. This is not to say you should not seek the option of IVF; what I am saying is that you need to look at your fertility support based on your whole health.

IVF used to be offered to women who married later and wanted to have a family right away. It was not as mainstream and not a developed industry because it was only available in some states and to people with means. Fertility clinics are busier than ever because they provide a baby making service and they will tell you if you wait that your chances of conception get lower and lower with each month that goes by. The fear of not being able to conceive is so great that doctors refer their young female patients to fertility clinics for egg freezing. The fear of not being able to have a baby fostered an entire campaign toward young women to freeze their eggs so they have some security in the future. There is no proof that a frozen egg from your younger self will be more viable than a fresh egg when you are older.

The point is that you have to look at the fertility industry as a health service "business," and with getting pregnant, you may feel like doctors know more about getting pregnant than you do, and you end up handing over your "free-will" and fertility to someone in a white coat because they point out one fact that you are over thirty-five years old. Fear is in the driver's seat and the hook is your age because you cannot deny that you are over thirty-five. This can cause you to continue to look for solutions based on your age. The solution you need to be searching for is not about age but how to optimize your fertility health.

I am not against fertility clinics; they help a lot of women and couples get pregnant. However, it is important is to make informed decisions based on facts that are relevant, and just being over thirty-five years old is not over the hill by any means.

Women have trouble getting pregnant at all ages. It just doesn't show up until you are ready to have a baby. In fact, many couples who are trying to conceive and have difficulty would have had difficulty even when they were younger; fertility was just not on their priority list.

Many young women are prescribed birth control in their teens and don't give fertility a second thought until they are in their thirties and want to have a baby. The problem with hormonal birth control is that it is an endocrine disruptor; it shares the same classification as pesticides. It intentionally interferes with your hormones by creating an imbalance that, in the end, affects the reproductive hormones and the ability to get pregnant. Being on an endocrine disruptor for years and years is not okay, and the answer is not to pump a woman with more hormones so she can get pregnant.

It was not that long ago that women had almost no control over their destinies, let alone their bodies. An unplanned pregnancy could derail the future of a college education, a career, or financial independence. There was a possibility you could end up marrying someone for security, endure shame from family and your community, or even be forced to give up the child for adoption.

Hormonal birth control offered, and still does offer, women freedom. The theme in women's health is that there is some underlying problem that can be solved by medicine, and that takes away your power. What is important to know is that you have control over your reproductive destiny, by understanding a little more about what is happening in your body and how hormones play this crucial role. Hormones are specialized chemicals and are part of the endocrine system.

The endocrine system is a chemical messenger system comprised of glands and organs that regulate the whole body; they release chemicals directly into the blood stream. We are most familiar with adrenal glands as they excrete adrenaline when we get stressed and will speed the heart rate and cause sweating, but any kind of disruption to the endocrine system causes the whole body to be in a state of constant low stress. There are many factors that can interfere with your body's health system and, in turn, affect fertility.

When researching fertility and getting pregnant over thirty-five, you may have discovered that there are a lot of the "statistics" about your chances of getting pregnant, such as at the age of thirty, you have a 20 percent chance of getting pregnant each month, but those chances dwindle over time so that by the time you reach forty, you have a 5 percent chance of success. When seeking help with fertility, it is challenging to ignore the age references. I can tell you that you have to know in your heart that it is not the case for you that your age will be an issue.

There are big lies, little white lies, and then there are statistics. Where is all this scientific and research evidence coming from? Shockingly, the statistics that are continually being used come from French birth records that are over three hundred years old. From 1670 to 1830, using church birth records, researchers came up with a statistic of how likely it would be for a woman over thirty to get pregnant. I'm not sure why data was collected from these churches or what women in seventeenth-century France have to do with women in the twenty-first century. Fertility was an issue in seventeenth-century Europe if you were looking for a male heir.

Somehow, the belief that women are considered a form of livestock to breed echoes. Unfortunately, continued "scientific" models and approaches to fertility are based on numbers that are not even relevant, and we have to take into consideration that science is still dominated by the male viewpoint. If we agree, we buy into a lie. So, stop googling statistics! If you think you are too old every time you google fertility statistics for women over thirty-five, you are going to get numbers that are three hundred years old.

I can't help but feel there is a continued lie being told to women, and that is that they are not powerful and don't know how their bodies work. Women are told there is always something wrong with them. What makes women different from men is that we, by design, have this "God" power – *Goddess* power – to create life. A woman's body has something known in Chinese medicine as an extraordinary vessel; it is the uterus and a special pathway called the *Bao Mai*. In women's bodies we have areas that are energy centers; in yoga practice, they can be referred to as chakras. What may be described as emotional, such as the feeling in your chest that you call love or sadness, from an energetic perspective, it is more than physical. Coming from a belief that we are more than our physical bodies, our thoughts move energy that in turn move the physical matter. The Bao Mai is an energy pathway that connects our "hearts" and uteruses with its magic. Our energy, or life force, has a very profound influence on our health and wellness. I more than believe that when we want to get pregnant, we connect our energy to the energies of the Universe (God or Goddess) to open that spirit pathway so that the spark of life can be ignited and then held.

What is not understood is often ridiculed or devalued. Age is a way to get into your psyche and tap into your feelings of unworthiness or brokenness. This attitude is still around, and unfortunately, you may feel like somehow it is your fault you can't get pregnant and look at your age as evidence. However, if a sixty-seven-year-old woman can have a baby, being over thirty-five is not what you should focus on.

There's a lot of data that we are consuming about infertility that is tailored to the female consumer. This is because women take the lead in figuring out why they are not getting pregnant; much of the material is directed toward women. The articles, the chat rooms, the newsletters, and ads for fertility clinics focus more on women having some problem. Material on male infertility is consumed by women, and it is the women who will initiate diet changes and make appointments for sperm analysis. First and foremost, a woman will assume that she has the problem and take on the burden of trying to solve it, exhausting every avenue related to female infertility. Women tend to consult and look for health solutions much more than men, so it is no surprise that much of fertility speaks to women solving their problem.

The male factor accounts for 40 to 50 percent of all infertility problems that couples have with conception, but the reality is that a man will not get a fertility checkup until the woman has gone through a battery of tests with the initial assumption that there is a problem with her reproduction.

Fertility is *big business*, and you have to ask if the data presented to you, so nicely packaged *conventional* wisdom, truly is wisdom or if it might be a money-sucking industry taking advantage of your desire to have a baby. If you have been researching, or if you have even been to a fertility clinic, the news is usually pretty dim. Those statistics from the 1600s come out along with statistics of having maternal illnesses or a baby with Down syndrome or other birth defects because you are old. If you go to a traditional fertility clinic, you will be offered hormones and will get the talk about age and fertility; you will feel urgency that there is not enough time or that it is too late for you. Here is where the adage of "if your only tool is a hammer, everything looks like a nail" comes into play. At least, fertility clinics will look at you from that perspective, and the doctors will convince you that you could be a nail, and if you agree, they will gladly hammer you.

This is why you may be getting the same information over and over again that when you are over thirty-five years old your ability to get pregnant goes down, but as a reminder, these are statistics, not your personal numbers.

At one point, I also had not questioned the idea of being too old, but the more women I saw and the evidence that kept showing up in my office to counter that assumption made me question the validity of all those statistics. It was when I met this woman named Gina that it became clearer to me that much of the way women were being treated in fertility clinics was in contrast to health and healing.

Gina came to me to be treated with acupuncture and herbs for fatigue and back pain. She was a single mom and forty-five years old. I was surprised when she shared that her daughter was a two-and-a-half-year-old toddler. I replied, "Oh," and I looked on her chart to check if she had a C-section. I also double checked that her age was indeed forty-five. I asked her if she had done IVF, and she said no.

Gina shared with me that she had read a book about a woman who had tried to have a second child and had been rejected by fertility clinics because she was aging out. The book was somewhat of a memoir/personal diary, and in it, the woman described her journey of going from fertility clinic to fertility clinic and being rejected because of her age and her hormone levels. The woman in the book underwent a radical change in her whole diet, drinking lots of wheat grass, increasing her exercise, and improving her outlook on her journey. I recognized the doctors in the book; though the names were changed, I knew who she was talking about just by hearing the name of the clinics and doctors' initials. I had also heard similar stories from my own patients who visited those same clinics on their fertility journey. The feedback was that they were "too old" and had poor-quality eggs and that if they wanted a baby, they needed to do IVF.

What was significant with Gina was that she did not go to a clinic and decided that she would implement changes in her diet and exercise, track her cycle, and try getting pregnant with her boyfriend, with the mind-set that if it happened, great. As it happened, she did get pregnant and delivered a happy and healthy baby. What I want to bring to your attention is that Gina had not sought fertility treatments at any clinic; therefore, her age factor and success would not be reflected in any statistics that fertility clinics use. I then thought there must be other women who conceive naturally and are in their late thirties and even early forties who are not being counted.

As we get older, does getting pregnant get more complicated? It can, but it still does not mean you are too old; it has a lot to do with how healthy we are. Fertility health is related to overall health, and individually, it will be important to address any underlying health issues, no matter what they are. When thinking about your fertility, remove age as the defining factor and you will be able to focus on what is important for your fertility health. Your body is in a constant state of transformation, and you have the opportunity every single day to improve your health so that you can get pregnant and have a happy and healthy baby. Your whole health counts.

This focus on being too old is a big obstacle, which is why it has its own chapter. There are other obstacles that show up to pull you off course, discourage you, and make getting pregnant a struggle. In the next chapter, we will cover removing those obstacles that you might not even be aware are working against you.

6

REMOVING THE OBSTACLES

ave you ever wanted something so badly that you did everything possible to get it? After trying everything and giving it your 110 percent effort, when that doesn't seem to work, you put more and more effort into it. Getting pregnant and having a baby has eluded you, even when you are doing everything right. It can make you want to tear your hair out, jump off a bridge, or peel your skin off your body. This is what I call "failing and flapping your wings at the same time but not getting to where you want to be."

In Chapter 4, we covered that big *why* and got clarity on how important it is to have a clear desire and purpose of this big and beautiful goal. A huge element of getting pregnant is developing the "fertility mind-set." This is prioritizing your focus on getting pregnant and becoming a mother. If you are feeling a bit confused, this is normal. Wanting and prioritizing need to be in alignment.

Women like yourself who come to me have this one thing in common: they are busy, busy, busy with the demands of a career, home, relationships, and leadership, and "adding" having a baby adds another source of stress. As busy women, taking on a lot of responsibilities is what we do. We handle it; we work later and harder, getting paid less money and squeezing everything into our schedules, and when all else fails, we give up the exercise class and work over the weekend to meet deadlines. We rearrange our schedules to accommodate family, friends, work events, vacations, projects, house cleaning, meetings, volunteering, fundraising, washing the car, and caring for pets and plants. When it comes time to get pregnant, we are juggling so much already that adding another plate is just not possible, but we still do it because that is what we do!

Everything you do is important and must be done; giving something up is not an option, and that is what makes this all so difficult, especially because it feels like you have no choice. These days just about everything has a sense of urgency, and it is easy to confuse this urgency with it being a priority. What comes to mind are those instant messages and texts that pop up and get your attention. Emails that have subject lines of "last chance" or the "doors are closing" to get you to pay attention because it's *urgent*. But it is not urgent for you; in fact, it is a distraction.

Let's say one day you would like to retire in Tuscany where you can live part of the year enjoying the Italian countryside with trips into Florence, to the bakery to get the artisanal bread, and to medieval towns where you can invite friends to stay. What this means is that if you want to do this when you retire, you would need to start putting a little bit of money aside consistently for this goal. It could be fifty dollars per week – that is about two Starbucks coffees a day. The urgency for saving the money will not necessarily be there because the goal is far in the future, but putting fifty dollars every week into your Tuscany fund is a priority for your retirement.

If you want to have a baby, then getting pregnant is the priority. What may show up as urgent, such as working late on deadlines, business meetings, or obligations to other people are no longer *the* priority. Although they may seem important, you cannot let them interfere with your goal of having a baby. Urgent activities will need to be reevaluated by comparing them to activities that may not have urgency but are a priority for your health, such as going to restorative yoga, sleep, eating healthy foods, and creating boundaries.

At one point, rescheduling appointments because of work travel, demands from bosses, and working on weekends might have been okay because your work was a priority. This is not to say you have to quit your job and that none of those things are important, but you should look at all those commitments and really look at which ones are going to get you to your goal of getting pregnant. They need to be put in the context of your priority is; all those other things are less important.

Urgency is not a priority. Priorities are important and need your attention always.

Looking backward, if you were twenty-five years old, you wouldn't have decided to get pregnant sooner because that would have thwarted your studies and the career you have. Your priority was different, as were the actions you took. It's just that you were never told that your fertility was a priority, even if you were not planning on having children for another decade or more. This is because there was no urgency; age made it so it was far in the future, and it was hard to imagine you might one day be confronted with that scenario.

The past is without the answers we need for now, though there are clues there for how we can approach getting pregnant and having a baby.

Sacrifice is something that plagues us; I personally don't think the idea that you have to give up one thing for another is a good thing, and that is not what a fertility mind-set is. However, what if you gave something up that you didn't want?

You are not being asked to stop working, even if that might have crossed your mind; it often does show up. You may feel like your whole life is on hold anyway as you focus on getting pregnant, but that does not work because it is about that energy of "having" to "do" more or "give up" something.

Sacrifice is the energy of losing out no matter which way you turn, and this causes more conflicting feelings and a feeling that things are out of control and you have no choice. I mentioned the saying "the way we do anything is how we do everything." If we have the mind-set and energy of sacrifice when it comes to having a baby, that is the way we will continue to approach this goal. It will exhaust the mind, body, and spirit. Having a baby is a beautiful goal, and it is important to hold this with *joy*. The fertility mind-set is about making fertility your priority, so it is on the top of your list. It's about time, and it is about energy and vision! The fertility mind-set is a way to get out of negativity and that stuck feeling, so you have a plan of action and clear steps to take while having everything managed. The Chinese proverb "a plan without action is a dream, action without a plan is disaster" sums this up well.

Before we continue, there is an exercise I want you to do. You will create a vision board on Pinterest. On that board you will create the life you envision for yourself with your baby. Everything goes on it – images of how you will feel, where you will live, the car you will drive, the vacations you will take, the foods you will eat, the games you will play, the baby clothes you will buy, and the holidays and birthday parties you will celebrate. Include all the things that you want your life to be and why you want this baby. I suggest that your husband or partner create a vision board, too, and you can share them.

First, I really like to do the individual ones – so there is no holding back or judgment – and then I suggest doing one together. I found that sometimes couples have different ideas of what life would be like with a baby, and together it can be even greater. With one couple, the husband envisioned sailing and living abroad and the wife had pictures of a house with a white picket fence, but when she saw travel adventure as a possibility that the family could share, she also wanted to have it as part of their combined vision board.

I promise this is not another physics example, though quantum physics explains a lot about confronting problems in life with just the right amount of zen to not put you off! With fertility and having a baby, you need to look at the time you are choosing to spend with *joy* and put that toward this project. It is not the same as renovating your kitchen or buying a pair of shoes. When you are in a place of *joy* and excitement, you are also in flow and alignment with your goal of having a baby. This means looking at the next six months to a year and clearing your calendar of the stuff that is not a priority.

At the end of this chapter, I will give you an exercise to help get clear on where you can release a lot of things you are doing that maybe you don't "need" to be doing. But for now, there are many things that seem to grab our attention, like Facebook and YouTube videos, scrolling through Instagram, or binging Netflix, and those things easily take over if you don't have boundaries around how you spend your time and "energy." With Netflix, it's hard to pull away, but it is an energy suck. Boundaries are important so that urgent stuff does not show up and steal and squash your dreams because you get pulled off your priority.

Things that are "urgent," like text messages and work emergencies, are not always a priority and need to be weighed in on if they will contribute to you getting pregnant and having a baby. If they are stressing you out, it is a good clue that it is not contributing to your goal of getting pregnant; energetically, it is sucking your life force. Take a hard look at what you commit to, and the time you have is a matter of efficiency as well. For example, Anne was an only child and had two parents who were getting on in age; they had her when they were a bit older, and now she is thirty-nine and her parents are in their late seventies. She was very involved with their care, and even though her partner was supportive, with elderly parents, the burden is usually on the child of the parents. Her father was showing early signs of Alzheimer's, and her mom was not fully cable of dealing with the situation. Anne was a kind of superwoman, running her business, checking in on her parents, doing food shopping, going over bills, and taking her parents to doctor appointments. This was a difficult situation because not only was it stressful, everything seemed to be a priority and urgent because she was their only child. Something had to be taken off her plate without sacrificing the care of her parents. It may seem obvious what she could do, but when she was "involved" as the point person for her parents, it didn't seem like she had options. The problem was that she did not even have a day off to be able to take a vacation let alone have a baby of her own.

If she would have looked at the whole picture and created a plan and schedule, there would suddenly be space for her and for her to have a baby. There were many things that she personally was doing for her parents that she really did not need to do, such as grocery shopping and going over bills; in fact, it was much more efficient to delegate those things. In her business, she delegated ordering supplies to the office manager and used a bookkeeper and a bill-paying service.

This marked the beginning of her relationship with Fresh Direct, a food market delivery service. She set up an account and worked with a caregiver to make sure that shopping was done and delivered. Several hours per week were now freed up and she could breathe. This also meant that when she spent time with her parents, it was quality time, not scrambling to fill the fridge.

Unfortunately there are people that can be in your life that keep you in holding patterns that suck your energy. You just don't normally see it because it's been there for a long time and it's a dynamic that is hooked in. But wanting to have a baby is something that will cause an energy shift, or I should say an energy shift has to happen so that a baby (new energy) can come in. This is a deep dive into aligning that *why* you want to have a baby and those dreams with actually removing things that are getting in the way of them. This will energetically open positive space so you can create that baby. Here's a secret – this is also a feng shui, which we will discuss in more detail in Chapter 11!

You have to take a look at your long list of "must dos" and "have to dos" and ask if everything on those lists deserves to be there. This does not mean that those things on the list don't have to get done. Instead, what I am offering up is whether you personally have to do them. I'll bet there are a bunch of things on your "to do list" and "must do list" that someone else could do and you can hand off those responsibilities to someone else. With women, there are usually a lot of house-related responsibilities that we are not willing to give up. It is also a bit of a trap that we fall into the females-as-nurturers role.

My patient Suzanne wanted to have a baby. Her husband was a little older and somewhat traditional in the sense that he did not intuitively volunteer to do house chores, food shopping, or laundry. She worked a full-time job and was getting her master's degree. The couple had been married for some time, and they waited before starting a family. Her husband worked from home while she commuted into the city, and when she got home, she would cook, clean up, do homework, and so on. They were pretty happy. When they struggled with getting pregnant, Suzanne made all the doctor appointments, did the testing searches online, and took on the burden of getting pregnant with a husband in tow. Not much changed schedule-wise or stress-wise for her husband, but for Suzanne, adding in doctor appointments, checking insurance, and tracking her cycle pushed her stress to where her hair was thinning and she was not getting enough sleep.

When Suzanne came to see me, one of the first things we worked on was to clear her schedule so that she could breathe. This may sound obvious, but if you are used to doing everything because it is easy for you to do and it only takes ten minutes here and fifteen minutes there, you have to look at releasing those things.

Now this was simple but not easy. Having someone do things for you can bring up resistance and may seem unnecessary, but your time and attention toward getting pregnant is a priority. So any time you can have someone else do something for you, do it.

Now, when I worked with Suzanne, the conveniences that we have today such as Amazon or Fresh Direct were not as developed, and perhaps that would not have made a difference where she lived. We've grown up with being self-sufficient, and we just like to do our own shopping, our own laundry, or clean our own houses, but it is not something that you *have* to do.

When we looked at Suzanne's time and how it was filled with chores that would stress her out if they were not done, we had to find a solution so that the house would be clean. The dynamic in Suzanne's relationship with her husband had to shift just a little. She communicated with him about what she needed, and while he grumbled a bit, he did not object.

What I have found is that because the fertility issue always seems to fall on the woman, often communication on what is needed falls a little by the wayside. Creating a partnership in the home environment is also setting up a support system. It can be easy for some couples to fall into traditional roles where the man makes more money and the woman then makes up the difference with more household responsibilities.

What it came down to was looking at the logistics and making agreements on what had to happen in order for her to relieve her stress, so they could focus on getting pregnant. Suzanne's husband didn't like the idea of a cleaner coming into the house when no one was there, so there was a compromise that a cleaner would come when someone was home. Was Suzanne happy about it? To be honest, not completely, but getting pregnant and having a baby meant much more than cleaning the house. Suzanne and her husband were definitely happy someone was cleaning their house when they had a baby!

Things like household chores and grocery shopping are the invisible things that take attention away from what your priority is, and that is holding that smiling baby in your arms nine months from now. Looking at six to twelve months as a timeline will give you space to put into practice what will improve your fertility health and also carries over through pregnancy. Planning out your time and energy will make all the difference.

Women take on way more than ever and multitask because we do it so well; we just keep on going and don't know when to stop. Why stop at all? It makes us feel accomplished. It is a strange phenomenon that seems to be the one area where women will be flexible for everyone else except for themselves. They are task masters and judges! Not only is this important to look at now, but it will definitely be the case once you have a baby!

EXERCISE: REPLACING THE "MUST" AND "HAVE" WITH "WANT" AND "WILL"

In this exercise, make a list of everything on your to-do list:

- On this list check off what is a must be done, taking into consideration what is a priority.
- You want to put an extra star next to the activities that are a priority.
- If there is anything that is *not* a must, put a little dot or *x* next to it
- On the list, mark what only you can do (highlight it so it stands out for you)
- Whatever is on the priority list, but not in the "only you can do," can be delegated or outsourced

- Then, get your calendar out and schedule the priority
  activities

This is a great activity to do with your partner or spouse, so you have a unified front. After you have your baby, it will be easier to organize around priorities of parenting. Infertility is very stressful on couples, and little things like laundry or dinner, meeting friends, or vacation plans can become sources of friction. By removing those invisible obstacles and getting clear about what is important (priority) for the success of getting pregnant, the feelings of struggle and difficulty will dissolve. You can then focus on the steps for success of getting pregnant.

In the next chapter, we will be reviewing some biology and physiology of the menstrual cycle and how to know when your most fertile time is. I will keep the information very basic, so we don't get lost in too much "scientific" jargon that then becomes confusing. The purpose is for you to be informed and not get overwhelmed.

7

THE TRUTH IS OUT THERE

You need to be informed about your health and make sure that you have checked all the boxes so that you have the whole picture of where you are in space and time. We are going to go over some basics about your biology and what the basic tests are so that you can develop a better relationship and understanding with your body's function and cycle, and you will learn how you can gather information about your cycle. To track your menstrual cycle, you might be using an app, or you may feel you already "know" when your cycle comes, but this is one of those times that I ask you to lean in and not check out.

LOOKING AT NUMBERS (WITHOUT STRESSING OR MAKING UP MEANING)

As we approach some of the biology of your body, it is easy to get triggered and start to worry about the "numbers" and then jump to despair about numbers meaning you can't get pregnant or that you are too old. Numbers and hormone levels are information that is gathered at a particular moment in time to help observe how your body is working. As a reminder, we are in a continuous dynamic state with our bodies' systems overlapping and influencing each other. With this topic I cannot tell you what your levels "should" be or what decisions you need to make for your situation. It is all too easy to stress over getting tests done. I think we all have some test anxiety that we will be labeled as not smart or defective, but making informed decisions about your health from a place of empowerment is what I support.

I want to bring you back to your priority of having a baby. This means gathering information so you can make informed decisions and take action. I am assuming that if you are reading this book, you have been to a doctor and gotten some preliminary blood tests done relating to hormones and fertility, such as follicle stimulating hormone levels, luteinizing hormone levels (if you have ovulated), your anti-Mullerian hormone levels, and your estrogen and progesterone, as well as thyroid and insulin resistance, and had gynecology exams to check for polyps, fibroids, and endometriosis.

It is important that you have these preliminary tests done to check hormone levels. Ask your primary care physician to do these tests for you or write a referral to have them done. This is information; it is not a life sentence or a judgment. Testing is not about finding what is wrong; it is about looking for what you can improve and make some small changes that will make great pivots. If your thyroid levels are a little low and the doctor prescribes thyroid medication to help you, this is a good thing. You can also look at what foods are in your diet that might be causing inflammation. Inflammation affects your thyroid functioning and we also know that this is information about your whole health, not just a gland in your body. Many women have thyroid problems that are subclinical and when they test for thyroid it comes back as being in normal range. Normal range is about a standard number that is applied to the general population. What we want to look at is what is *true* for you.

There are two types of attitudes I've observed in people who struggle with health issues and fertility. The first are patients believe that a doctor or the medical system will save them and blindly accept whatever from a white coat and stethoscope as the gold standard and do not seek a second opinion. They believe wholeheartedly that someone else knows more about their body and that's it. When I encounter people who rely on their doctors to fix them, I notice they are usually not proactive with their health and eventually are on three to five medications for conditions that are preventable by lifestyle changes. Obviously, this is not you, or you would not be reading this book. The other attitude is one where a patient never goes to a doctor and they don't believe in Western medicine. Being healthy and improving fertility health does not work well with either extreme. It is best to look at all the ways you can be supported and what the best way will be for you.

If you struggle with weight and have difficulty losing weight unless you diet intensely, exercise, and eventually can shed a few pounds only to yo-yo back to the same weight or even more, the conclusion is *not* that you are undisciplined or lazy. There is most likely some underlying metabolic dysfunction that is not being picked up, and it is something *small* that is out of your awareness and considered insignificant on tests. The good news is that it is a big *clue* for you to look at other areas of your life and health that have not gotten attention.

Having a test come back as normal is a blessing and a curse. In some cases, you might have wanted to get a diagnosis so that you would *know* what is wrong, but if it is "normal," the diagnosis is usually "unexplained infertility," which can cause more anxiety and cause more anxiety along the lines of "what is wrong with me?"

There is nothing "wrong" with you; your body is in a dynamic process and understanding a bit more about our biology will reveal that you are "normal."

REPRODUCTION BASICS

What is important is that you get a refresher about the birds and the bees. The last time most women heard about it was when they were in middle school and had sex education class. I don't think anyone was interested in the biology part of the lecture, and I think that the instructors don't want to encourage too much "learning" on that subject. It seems to be uncomfortable for all adolescents as their bodies are developing and they feel self-conscious and ashamed. You may also be feeling a weird shame about your reproduction, and it can make you feel uncomfortable. This is completely normal. It is not a matter of being stupid or smart; unless you are a biologist or work in fertility, most people are amazed when they learn about how reproduction works.

For the patients in my office, I do a brief overview of the reproductive cycle and then we look at details as they relate specifically to their body and cycle. I'm providing that same overview here for you, just as if you were sitting in front of me as one of my patients.

Women have a twenty-eight-day biological cycle. If you ever wondered why women are associated with the symbol of the moon, this is because of the twenty-eight-day "moon" cycle. When figuring out what day of your cycle you are, the first day is the day that you bleed. The bleeding is not so much blood as it is the shedding of the lining of the uterus, and it coincides with a drop in hormones (progesterone). This is normal if you are not pregnant, so the body signals to start over.

The bleeding will last from two to seven days, and while your body is cleaning out the dead tissue, a follicle/s (egg) is maturing in your ovaries in response to a stimulating hormone (FSH). When the follicle reaches a certain size or maturity, another hormone is released (LH) to direct the egg to leave the ovary, marking ovulation. This is around mid-cycle and can be day twelve to sixteen, but it can also be a little earlier or later.

The egg then makes its way through the fallopian tube toward the uterus where it will encounter sperm. The sperm will try to penetrate the surface of the egg to fertilize it; not just any sperm can do it; in fact, hundreds of millions of sperm are trying to penetrate the egg surface for a chance to pass on genetic information to the one egg. Once a sperm has passed through the surface, no other sperm can penetrate and the exchange of genetic material starts and the egg develops into a zygote. Over seven to nine days this zygote continues to develop and implant on the lining of the uterus that has been thickening with healthy tissue, and the cells emit a hormone (HCG), which is what a pregnancy test measures is present.

This process has several steps and interruptions can occur at many points of the process. I would like to add that only one in a million sperm will be able to get within range of the egg during this natural process. The thing about salmon swimming upstream is they first have to get there.

I have included a link to a simple overview of reproduction from Khan Academy so that you can get reacquainted with basic anatomy, physiology, and biology. The more you learn about the body, the more informed you will be and, in turn, be able to discern whether something feels right: https://www.khanacademy.org/science/high-school-biology/hs-human-body-systems/hs-the-reproductive-system/a/hs-the-reproductive-system-review

I call this "doing some homework."

BASIC CHECKLIST TO RULE OUT COMPLICATIONS

Methodically and logically, you need to go through the process of elimination of possible obstacles and get them tested.

I like to start by asking if there is a physical obstruction. Is there something that is blocking the egg from going down the fallopian tube and meeting the sperm? If you are trying to get to a destination, the main road is easiest or the path of least resistance. For some reason, this is not the first test that is done, but in my personal opinion, it is the logical thing to look at.

At this point, I will assume that you have most likely heard of a hysterosalpingogram (HSG). HSG is an X-ray procedure used to see whether the fallopian tubes are patent (open) and if the inside of the uterus (uterine cavity) is normal. HSG is an outpatient procedure that usually takes less than five minutes to perform. There are many women who may have "irregular" cycles but that doesn't matter so long as the egg can meet the sperm. Making sure that the tubes are clear is a no brainer.

When trying to get pregnant and have a baby, you need an egg, sperm, and a uterus; those are the main ingredients and those you have. So, at the same time that you are checking whether you have any obstructions have your spouse or partner get their sperm checked too. Forty to 50 percent of infertility is related to male infertility. Having a sperm analysis done is not an invasive procedure, and it can be done at a clinic.

Culturally, our masculinization of men creates a tendency to ignore aches and pains. They are taught to suppress feelings both emotionally and physically and, therefore, are not as disciplined as women in getting regular checkups. It is common for men to develop a varicocele on their testicles, which impedes blood flow and can cause low sperm production and morphology. In our computer age, there is a lot of sitting and it is pretty common and should be checked. Most procedures for women are much more invasive, so it makes sense to do the checkups and testing that are the easiest, least costly, and most accessible first.

I know that you may feel some resistance to getting tests because when you had them, they brought up immense feelings of shame and you didn't even want to look at them. There is a negative connotation with tests. But you should take advantage of the information, as it will help you like a puzzle missing a small piece to complete the picture.

Why we have resistance to testing comes from when we were students and taking exams. Questions may not have seemed fair. Maybe it felt like you were being judged on how smart you were. The difference is that this testing is about gathering basic information, and it will help you.

RELATIONSHIP WITH YOUR DOCTORS AND HEALTHCARE PRACTITIONER

It is *very* important that you find doctors and practitioners who you have a relationship with – ones who you have access to, return your calls, answer your questions, and who you *trust*. Doctors are human; they know what they know, and while they have information that you may not have, they also have their limitations. A physician who without judgment encourages you to get *healthy* and explore other ways of improving your health helps empower you to seek solutions for your health.

We can't help but care what doctors say because they hold positions of power. I have found that doctors who express openness to other forms of healing, even if they don't necessarily understand or personally believe them, gain respect and trust from their patients.

Some doctors will tell you not to do something because it is not scientifically proven or something that they believe in, and that is the same with every person you encounter. They can help you as far as *they* believe it is possible and not what is *true* for you. I believe that we are ever evolving, and one direction is not going toward decline but evolving, and there are opportunities to get healthier always in front of us. When one thing seems to be blocked, life moves to open another to get through.

The difference in your chances of getting pregnant is like night and day when you work with someone who cares about you. They will also encourage you and support you, because in the end, they want you to be holding a healthy and happy baby in your arms.

ELIMINATING INFLAMMATION

Another obstacle to fertility that is so prevalent in modern society, although often overlooked, is underlying inflammation. This comes in the form of exposure to plastics, chemicals, and pesticides that are endocrine disruptors, and it is especially the case for women with a history of long-term hormonal birth control use.

Looking at a whole health history, there are a couple of things that will pop out, and one of them is hormonal birth control. Hormonal birth control is considered an endocrine disruptor and if you were on birth control for any period of time, your body will need to detox itself. The body is in a constant state of moving toward health by metabolizing nutrients and eliminating waste and toxins. When there is a buildup of toxins and hormones in the body, if they cannot be eliminated, they need to go somewhere they will not cause a major disruption to the body's homeostasis. They then get stored in places like the liver or in body fat. Common symptoms are gas, bloating, extra weight around the middle, and some skin sensitivity and allergies. After years of exposure to these endocrine disruptors, the residual toxins in the body cause inflammation and will need to be detoxed from your body.

By eating more plant based and organic foods, you don't have to process the chemicals that are in processed foods. This allows your body to naturally eliminate any excess toxins that were stored. This detox will make a big difference with overall health and fertility because the inflammation is reduced.

Endocrine disruptors are chemicals, both natural and man-made, that mimic or interfere with the body's hormones, known as the endocrine system. Because these chemicals interfere with our own endocrine systems, they can cause developmental, reproductive, brain, and immune problems. These hormone disruptors are found in many everyday products, including some plastic bottles and containers, liners of metal food cans, detergents, flame retardants, food, toys, cosmetics, and pesticides.

Exposure to these chemicals also can cause chronic yeast infections. Some women get yeast infections every month as they cycle, and they end up taking antibiotics. Then, the following month, they get one again. Women are also triggered by stress. So, the cycle of antibiotics can cause more imbalances in the body, preventing the yeast from ever truly going away; it just recedes and waits for the next opportunity to grow back. This is what causes a lot of underlying inflammation, and women can go for years having recurring episodes.

With of the use of antibiotics, there is most likely a gut imbalance that can then contribute to overall body inflammation. My recommendation is to look at addressing this inflammation not for a short period of time but consistently. This is where a doctor might suggest you take a probiotic for a month or so, like a drug, but the truth is, gut health plays a key role in immune function as well as brain chemistry and hormones. Making sure that your gut and intestinal flora are healthy is an ongoing health maintenance.

Even *if* you are planning to go through IUI or IVF, being in the best of health is what you need to do. Taking fertility hormones has risks and eliminating health issues in advance will increase your chances of success. That is what we are looking for.

THE MENSTRUAL CYCLE

Tracking your menstrual cycle is the biology of reproduction. This is what will give you an idea of what is going on in your own body; think of it as a biological diary. For example, what happened this morning? You might write, "Day 1 – my temperature is 98.2 degrees Fahrenheit, some spotting and cramping, a bit of loose bowels, and I feel a bit weepy."

I like to have my patients' charts. It is a great way to be productive and gather information that is useful, no matter what your next steps will be for getting pregnant. This will be useful if you have a timeline of when you are planning to start on a cycle, I found that the charts are evidence of hormonal fluctuations that are not picked up on tests.

With fertility testing, they usually ask, "How long is your cycle?" If it is twenty-eight days, the assumption is that you ovulate in the middle of the cycle, but that is not always the case, so by recording your temperature first thing every morning before getting out of bed and then noting cervical mucus consistency when you go to the bathroom, you will be able to have much more accurate information about your body's cycle. This way, you will know your body and its rhythm and feel the changes of when your most fertile time is. Self-knowledge will help you make informed decisions about what is right for you.

Body temperature can fluctuate depending on weather or even moving a lot can make your temperature go up before you take it; also if you have a cold or allergies your temperature will be affected. However, we are looking at the big picture and collecting data.

Ovulation sticks record whether your body releases LH to direct ovulation. I recommend using ovulation sticks on day ten of your cycle until you get a positive line so you will be sure to record the data. What I have found with some women is that their cycle may vary from month to month; stress can cause a cycle to be shorter or longer. All this is information that will help you. I will include a link to the ovulation chart for tracking your cycle I use with my patients and you are welcome to use it too.

It is available on my website at this link: https://www.integrativehealingarts.com/intake-forms.

Further, here is an example of how getting the right tests helped to heal an underlying health condition that could be addressed, so one of my patients could get pregnant. Marta and her husband had been married for less than a year. She was thirty-nine when she met Kevin on a blind date that she was originally not going to even bother going to. She thought that the time for her to marry and have children had already passed, but their relationship moved quickly; within ten months, they were married. Having a baby was what they both wanted.

They immediately sought assistance from a fertility clinic as Marta was already forty. Marta also came to get treated with acupuncture, as she was dedicated to doing everything she could to increase her chances of getting pregnant and having a healthy pregnancy. Marta was heavy, though she exercised regularly, she ate clean (she was mostly plant based), slept well, and was healthy, but no matter what she did, she could not lose weight. She was at least fifty pounds overweight, placing her in the obese category. She was tired a lot, but this could be explained by having a demanding job and, like most people, didn't have boundless energy. So none of these symptoms seemed to be a concern for the fertility clinic. Being overweight can be an indication of PCOS or other metabolic imbalances that can cause problems with fertility, including miscarriage.

When we went over the checklist of tests that were done, there were some that seemed to be missing, in particular a thyroid test. Humans are animals, and our bodies should be efficient and respond to the environment we are exposed to. So as the weather gets colder or the winter months come in, we will gain some weight. This is a natural response to store fat to keep us warm, and during the summer, we tend to lose weight. Extra fat and weight are not efficient; they take extra energy to carry around, and the fact is that we live in environmentally controlled temperatures and get a sufficient amount of food on a regular basis and therefore don't need all that extra weight. The excess indicates that there is something metabolically off and I shared this information.

Marta and her husband did not feel so confident working with the initial fertility clinic they chose, so I recommended they work with another reproductive specialists whom I had met in person and knew had compassion and a great reputation. I encourage all my patients to get second opinions about treatments and blood tests, especially if there is something that is off, so Marta got a full blood panel and made sure that all of her test results were recent and her gynecological exams were also current. Low and behold, there was something off with her thyroid, and the doctor had picked up some numbers that led her to figure out that her thyroid was low. This explained the difficulty with losing weight, and if it had not been picked up, all the fertility treatments that she was going to do might not have been effective, or she might have miscarried.

During the three months that it took to make sure her thyroid levels were stable, she lost weight, she was able to take that time to work on herself, and she also was charting her menstrual cycle and taking advantage of her most fertile days. The plan was that she would then go back to the clinic and start an IVF cycle. When her period did not come, she did a pregnancy test and found out that she and her husband had conceived naturally.

YOUR HEALTH KNOWLEDGE IS YOUR HEALTH POWER

The reason that learning about how *you* work health-wise is important because fertility is not just about reproduction; it is overall health. The fertility aspect is a door that we enter inside a big house. To get to the room, you need to know the schematics and how to get there. Often, fertility is referred to as a garden. You have to tend the soil and plant the seeds. If the soil has not been taken care of, it will be hard to grow the seeds into flowers and plants. Without getting informed about your body and your health, it is easy to feel ashamed because you lack knowledge, and that can make you believe that someone in a white coat will know more about *you* and what is right for *you*. This is where we can hand our power over and go back to being that twelve-year-old in sex education class who doesn't want to talk about what happens in her body. The shame will also keep you from seeking help or make you feel helpless and out of control.

This is where we gain knowledge without judgment. The moment we judge the information, we have committed ourselves to a story about the way it will end up. This can block our ability to see what options there are and the next steps are for us. Just as you are over thirty-five and keep looking for information about fertility for those who over thirty-five, you will end up getting answers that will cause you to jump to conclusions and feed your *fear* of being too old. The shame and guilt that comes up can be paralyzing and you need to know that this is also what may cause you to not want to look at your health because you will judge everything you did and then end up condemning yourself. Hopefully, this is not the case.

As a reminder, if you have a doctor, therapist, family member, friend, or someone similar who blames you or says things that are not helpful, such as, "Well, you should have done [blank] when you had the chance," this is not helpful. Looking at numbers takes courage; be willing to do the exercises and not judge them. You need to give yourself a few months of consistently tracking and making sure to schedule appointments and tests and chart them. After doing this, you will see an amazing collection and representation of a process.

Medication, such as birth control, is a red flag for me, especially when I see patients who were on it for some time, in some cases up to twenty years! This means that from the time they were a teenager, their body never had the chance to cycle naturally. Often, being on birth control can disguise underlying health conditions that show up later, such as endometriosis and PCOS.

Depression is one of the side effects of hormonal birth control and studies show an increase in prescriptions for mood stabilizers after several months on birth control. Women tend to be prescribed much more anti-anxiety medications, antidepressants, and antibiotics than men. Women are prescribed lots of drugs, and I have a big opinion about women's health. There is still the idea that women are emotional and weak and that giving us a pills will take care of the problems we experience without addressing the inequities and the stressors that we face. These are also environmental factors that we touched on in previous chapters regarding getting support and making choices on how to get it. There are many things that we cannot change about the outside world and about how people behave, and I want to bring this to your awareness so you don't fall into a pattern of self-blame or discouragement. Know thy enemy – ignorance.

We want to be clear about facts such as tests and measures and then use that information to make informed decisions about the best ways of addressing what is revealed. One of the challenges when we start looking at numbers and tests and trying to make sense of our biology is we can run into the idea of perfection. As women we try to do everything perfectly so we can control the outcome. But testing is also where you can make the most impact on your fertility and getting pregnant. In the next chapter, we will be exploring ways that you may be working against yourself and how you can learn to get out of your own way.

8

IS PERFECTION SABOTAGING YOU?

erhaps you have gone full on drill sergeant with yourself doing every possible healthy activity to get pregnant, yet you find yourself more and more stressed and further from the goal of having a baby. You avoid alcohol, caffeine, and seafood (mercury), and your diet consists of every recommendation you have read about. You're in fertility boot camp.

At some point, I was going to call the way of working with fertility and getting clear about it "fertility boot camp," but women were already putting so much pressure on themselves to do everything perfectly that this in itself becomes a source of stress. Our Western culture has an attitude toward the Earth – violent and destructive cultivation of the land, destruction of the ecosystem, and the use of chemicals and pesticides to augment production. This is very much the same approach with women and fertility.

The approach to women, fertility, and their bodies needs to change. You are already perfectly formed and are part of the natural order. You have this gift of creation inside of you, and the name of the program is called "The Fertility Goddess." If you have ever seen images of fertility goddess statues, they are quite round, not skinny like Barbie dolls. Women and their body image are in constant turmoil; just about every woman that you ask will tell you that she is fat or that there is something that needs work. So aside from striving for a kind of physical perfection, there is also striving to do fertility perfectly.

The one thing that causes a big problem is "doing everything perfectly." This is trying to fit into an ideal of what fertility health is. This is not to say to start smoking and drinking because it doesn't matter, because it does make a difference; however, the way you go about being vigilant and creating rules about what you can and cannot do will drive you crazy as the focus is on being perfect by some standard. This is trying to "fix" something that is "broken." You are not broken, so fixing is the wrong energy with regard to your mind, body, and spirit.

Your fertility health is your whole health, and understand that, as women, we have a cycle that ebbs and flows. It is referred to as a "moon cycle," and if you listen to your body, you will be able to work with it. If you have been "attacking" this "problem" the way you address other problems, you are missing this important part of your body, and you will be met with major resistance. If you feel like you are in a choppy sea trying to swim and are getting pulled down and tumbled around, like being in a washing machine, the first thing you need to do is stop fighting the current. Feel where it pulls you and use the energy of the current to push you back toward the shore.

We get so busy trying to do the "right thing" and do it perfectly that we fight our own bodies and expect them to submit. When they don't respond the way they are "supposed to" according to medical texts, it leads us to think we are broken.

After having some difficulty getting pregnant, most women will go the medical route and be given all kinds of health scenarios about what is wrong with them. As I mentioned, I definitely believe that we must do baseline tests because it is an extra way to cross-check what we are doing and improving on. However, I don't know any female over seven years old who doesn't have some self-criticizing thought. Women and girls think they are too fat, thin, short, or tall or have ears too big, hair too straight, hair too curly, eyes too small, nose too big, chin too weak, feet too big, hips too wide, boobs too small, buttocks too fat, thighs too fat, skin too pale, too many freckles, and on and on. That is why plastic surgery is a massive business.

Why do I bring this up? Because, from a young age, we, as women, are taught to not like ourselves and that we are flawed and imperfect. When we get all awkward and then our periods come, also known as "the curse," the beginning of puberty primes us for hating and rejecting what makes us nonmale. I'm guessing the idea of celebrating womanhood can make you cringe a bit because we are talking about bleeding every month – *ick*! If you are having these feelings around your body and how it is not cooperating with your plans, it is important to get to know yourself and your unique biology. The word for *female* in Tahitian, *wahine*, is the same as the word for *goddess*. The word *ugly* does not exist.

Looking at other cultures around the world, women are viewed as powerful because they have a menstrual cycle, even if they are suppressed. The restrictions placed on women in non-Western cultures have to do more about how they have been powerful and control men. Think about Helen of Troy. Think about women being persecuted as witches because of their power. However, in the West, the use of shame is what controls women and how they think of themselves.

Going back, the Tahitian word *wahine* demonstrates one of our greatest gifts that females possess – the creation of life. We are the vessel in which the spirit comes through into a physical being. So, what am I talking about? In the same way, you need to step into your power and learn what it is and how to use it.

A woman's biology and physiology have a cycle, which includes changes in hormones and metabolic processes, and adapting your lifestyle around your cycle, such as your diet, exercise, and activities, will help you balance energy and be in alignment with the natural biological rhythm of your body.

The menstrual cycle, or fertility cycle, is often referred to as a "moon cycle" because it is also a twenty-eight-day cycle and has four parts where there are hormonal changes, physical changes, and energy and emotional shifts. This means it is completely normal to not be the same perky personality and expect yourself to feel like everything is great all the time. Metabolically, there are shifts happening, so if you are not in the rhythm of understanding your body, you can become hard on yourself. This applies to focus at work and to relationships, socialization, the desire for certain foods, confidence, and vulnerability.

Here is a brief overview of what happens during the different phases of your cycle. You may have different experiences, and that is normal. The days may vary, as you may have a little longer cycle or shorter one, but that does not matter because you still cycle.

MENSTRUAL PHASE (APPROXIMATELY DAYS ONE TO SIX)

The menstrual phase is also known as the bleed (days one to six). The hormones of progesterone are low, as well as estrogen, and the lining of the uterus has disintegrated and sheds, causing bleeding. The body begins releasing follicle-stimulating hormones to wake up follicles in preparation of ovulation during day two and three of your bleed. Emotionally, you may feel vulnerable and can be weepy or feel anxious or down. It is common to get headaches or migraines, skin breakouts, loose stools, and some women get yeast infections or cold sores. Energy during this phase is at its lowest, and you may just feel like sleeping. You may have low iron and vitamin B.

THE FOLLICULAR PHASE (APPROXIMATELY DAYS SEVEN TO THIRTEEN)

During the first days of your period, you produce follicle-stimulating hormones that signal the follicles to respond and this overlaps with the menstrual phase. Post-period, the hormones of progesterone and estrogen are rising, and you may feel more alert and have better energy all around. This is during the time that the egg follicles are growing.

THE OVULATORY PHASE (APPROXIMATELY DAYS THIRTEEN TO TWENTY-ONE)

During this stage, estrogen peaks, testosterone and progesterone rise, and your body releases luteinizing hormone signaling ovulation. Women feel most attractive and have a higher sex drive during their ovulation phase. Energy is higher, and you may find you have better coordination. Emotionally, you may feel better about yourself and want more contact; this is also because you are fertile and that is part of nature's drive.

THE LUTEAL PHASE (APPROXIMATELY DAYS TWENTY-TWO TO TWENTY-EIGHT)

Post-ovulation, progesterone continues to rise, and the uterine lining thickens in anticipation of implantation (pregnancy). Estrogen will also rise. Emotionally, there can be mood swings such as irritability, weepiness, or both. Cravings for sugar and junk foods and water retention can start as well as breakouts, bloating, and constipation.

If pregnancy does not occur, the progesterone levels drop, and the uterine lining will start to disintegrate and eventually shed. Energy may feel erratic and you might bump into things. This is because the hormones can cause ligaments to be elastic and weaker so coordination can be clumsy.

You want to gather this information about your body with acceptance and love and not use it as evidence of imperfection. Recording your cycle and ebbs and flows in your energy, emotions, and physical changes is a way to have a stronger mind-body connection and to feel that you are in charge of your destiny.

CHARTING EXERCISE

If you have already been tracking your menstrual and ovulation cycle using an electronic monitor or phone app, I want you to start to use a thermometer, ovulation sticks, and a paper chart. Why is this? You may be asking yourself, "Why are we using charts, thermometers, and pee sticks when there are electronic monitors and fancy phone apps?" Here is a secret: electronics are a huge trigger for the stress response. Stress is one of the biggest barriers for conceiving, which you already know. Electronics and blue lights interrupt the circadian rhythm the body's biological clock that also regulates sleep and reproductive hormones. Therefore, we want to take the stress away from getting pregnant and not have it bundled with emails, texts, phone calls, and so on.

Manually taking your temperature first thing in the morning and charting is a way of focusing and creating a fertility mind-set. The fertility mind-set places you and fertility first. You are physically doing the process and creating a practice. The fertility mind-set is what creates perspective and sets the intention and the energy moving throughout the day.

As we have been looking at overall health and you look at how your body has a natural rhythm, you can start to manage your energy, keeping in mind that there are some times of the month when you will have greater mental acuity and can take on more. On the other hand, there will be other times when your body will need more rest, so honor that time by not forcing yourself to do more.

Here is a place where judgement and shame will come in. If you were able to do everything you wanted one week and felt accomplished, but the next week you could not repeat it, there are biological and metabolic factors at work. Women expect themselves to perform like men; this is where our ideas of how we should perform come from. I have to say, this is a ridiculous myth, as women have superpowers of their own. We have to look at the structure of society in the West, which was developed by men and for men over the past two thousand years. It is the dominant model, so in order for women to succeed in this model, they have to think and behave like men; however, this is not so natural for us, and we struggle. The point that I am making is that the expectation of fertility health comes from this model and perpetuates certain flawed standards and assumptions of how we should be in order to breed.

TOXIC PRODUCTS THAT AFFECT YOUR HEALTH AND FERTILITY

Many of the ways that women are regarded socially also drives them to look a certain way and meet an ideal. These activities cause women to believe that perfection is the standard in all areas, and if they are not getting pregnant, there is something that they are not doing perfectly. Women are so vulnerable to seeing perfection because it comes from an underlying idea that they are inherently flawed, and if they can conform to some ideal then they will be accepted. Some mommy support groups can turn into toxic environments for that reason and degrade to being a competition of who is more perfect. So much of what society expects form women and what they put themselves through to achieve an ideal are the very things that interfere with their hormones and fertility.

Much of what is advertised and marketed to women is not so healthy for them. Use of products, such as makeup, perfumes, hair products, soaps, shampoos, nail polish, and creams that may contain chemicals that are endocrine disruptors can cause problems with fertility. Household cleaners, plastic containers, and detergents also disrupt hormones. Sixty-six percent of women from the ages fifteen to forty-nine use hormonal birth control and twice as many women are on psychiatric medications compared to men. With all these products women are getting exposed to there can be an accumulation of factors that can pull your body off balance. You will need to take a look at products that are endocrine disrupting and begin to remove them; this is not only for fertility but also because these products are related to thyroid illness and increased cases of cancer as well.

Don't get too crazy but start to look at using glass containers instead of plastic. Read labels of personal care products such as makeup, deodorants, and shampoos that contain known endocrine disrupting chemicals such as phenols, parabens, and phthalates. Be more aware of any products that will be in contact with your food or directly on your body where chemicals can be absorbed. This will also be important for your spouse or partner as sperm can easily be affected as well. There are plenty of natural products that you can use, and I encourage you to look for ones you will like so that you can feel good about what you are consuming.

YOU ARE WHAT YOU THINK

The history of women being hysterical and overly emotional continues to permeate how women are treated in the world of medicine, and this is why you need to be aware of these influences, including how you think about your fertility health. This is why you need to be doing some "homework" around where you can make positive changes to your environment by eliminating as much exposure to chemicals as you can. Don't judge whether or not it is perfect; you are looking at the big picture. You are learning and being proactive.

When you started off, you might have gone "boot camp style," forcing yourself to make extreme changes to your diet, exercise routine, supplements, and scheduled time for sex. Maybe you held your legs in the air to eating pineapples. You also may wonder, "How do unhealthy women get pregnant, and I'm doing everything right and it's still not happening?" Don't start becoming unhealthy; there is something that you have been missing, and that is your whole health, not just focusing on your reproduction, which will also come in. What you have been told to focus on is inaccurate. As you start to put the puzzle pieces of your health rhythm together via your cycle, you can also use that knowledge to support your fertility naturally.

I recommend that you work with an alternative and Chinese medicine practitioner to help support your health naturally. This is also a window into where you can use some support with supplements, herbs, acupuncture, bodywork, and mind-body practices to boost your fertility.

Acupuncture is one of the most effective treatments for helping your body heal because it taps into the parasympathetic nervous system – the rest and digest mechanism. Studies show that certain neuropeptides are released that are the "feel-good" chemicals that give you an overall sense of well-being, and immune and healing mechanisms are also activated. I recommend getting acupuncture for overall well-being, and a skilled acupuncturist will also be able to support your fertility health. If you are afraid of needles, you can also receive acupressure, though it will be a little different.

Bodywork or massage stimulates your whole nervous system; the skin is the largest part of your brain. We tend to ignore how our body feels unless it is complaining and getting massages can help you become aware of where you hold tension and also where you may have energy blocks. Allowing someone to touch you is about being comfortable in your body and having trust. You can also get some reflexology or hand massage. Reflexology is based on a body mapping system where the hands and feet have points that reflect the whole body, so you can treat a back pain by pressing or massaging certain areas on the feet or hands. I recommend that you try some of these natural ways to support your health.

Mind-body practices involve intentional breathwork and connection to your body. Yoga and Tai Chi are forms of moving meditation. A mind-body exercise you can do first thing in the morning is to focus on breathing in and out while scanning your body, from your toes up to your head with each breath, clearing any thoughts that intrude while you do this exercise. What this does is help you to connect to your body and mind and helps you be in control of your nervous system, creating a habit of feelings of well-being. This will help you with having calmness throughout the day and not get pulled into unwarranted stress.

I cannot tell you specific herbs or supplements you should be taking because I don't have your specific health information in front of me, so it would be irresponsible on my part. However, what is important to be on the lookout for is if you find that you are not doing something the way you think you should or are worried about doing it perfectly, thinking there should be a specific outcome. You might be sabotaging your efforts.

Allow yourself to release your Goddess energy. You have to think of yourself like a *Goddess*. However, first you need to know what is going on in your body so you can make the best decisions for your fertility health so you can get pregnant and hold that happy, healthy baby in your arms.

In the next chapter, we will shed some light on some areas that are a blind spot for many; this has to do with beliefs and with people in our lives who create negative energy and block us. Becoming aware of some of these blind spots can be surprising, because they are often right under your nose.

9

UNLEARNING WHAT WE HAVE LEARNED

One of the biggest blocks to getting pregnant is battling the negative thoughts that come up and torture you. In the previous chapter we looked at the idea of perfection and those are beliefs that we learned and adopted or have been programmed into our psyches. The struggle that we experience is when what we have learned does not match the results that we are expecting. That is when the internal alarms go off and we experience pain and suffering. What is this struggle? It is the negative thought patterns that color reality and make our efforts seem like there is no hope. These thoughts are like that little devil sitting on your shoulder whispering in your ear negativity. Unfortunately, those voices seem to find evidence to make them seem true. So, as you move forward, even knowing that you are making the right decisions for your health and fertility, the old patterns will pop up, such as "but I am over thirty-five or over forty."

The struggle comes from creating meaning from the information you acquire and putting it through your own "filter of hell." This is when we pick out certain things or listen to problems and then overlay them onto our goal of becoming pregnant. How a woman thinks about herself and what she says to herself will influence her success. You may not realize that you do say things to yourself that are not helpful and can actually be damaging to your nervous system and physical body. These are part of deeper cultural patterns that come with being a woman and how we were raised.

In the case of fertility, having family members who got pregnant and had kids "easily" can cause you to think there is something wrong with you because you compare yourself to someone who you believe is "just like you." However, there is no one just like you. You are on a mission, and part of that mission has a purpose of becoming a mother; otherwise you would not be here right now. You are not broken, even if it feels that way.

No matter where you are in your journey, it will be essential that you have to take charge of those negative thought patterns and do a mind-set reset. If you keep asking yourself, "what is wrong with me?" you will undoubtedly come up with a bunch of answers to satisfy the question, but that does not mean that they are true.

A question causes us to look for an answer, but it also directs us to a kind of answer that will lead us back to a belief, so that it is a nice packaged, closed circuit. If you are not aware that you are doing this, when the opportunity and the answers you have been looking for show up, you will not see them. Instead, you will be looking for answers based on a flawed question. Once you develop the fertility mind-set, you will be able to recognize what is relevant for you and remove and replace the thoughts that don't help you with your priority of getting pregnant.

SELF-CULTIVATION TOOLS AND FENG SHUI

In East Asian medicine, we use many tools to help a person heal themselves. You might already be using many of these tools, such as doing yoga or being part of a book club, taking an art class, gardening, or volunteering for a cause. This comes from the idea of self-cultivation that we can expand our minds intellectually and have a healthy body and an environment that supports us and will improve our lives and those of our community. This comes from an understanding that we are all interconnected even if we cannot see it. Eating foods that are in season nourishes mindfulness, mind-body practices, exercise to move energy through the meridians (energy pathways) and breathing exercises that calm the nervous system and what is our environment.

If we can control our nervous system response, such as the fight or flight, we are able to become self-aware of what is influencing us. This is a practice of being able to respond versus react, and that is a choice. It is a way for the individual to become more aware of who they are and how they are in relationship to themselves and their family, community, country, and universe. This is self-awareness, and from an Eastern perspective, it is the road to enlightenment. You will need to be willing to break away from some of the patterns and thoughts that hold you back and make getting pregnant and having a baby so challenging.

One way that I have found very effective for breaking old patterns is through feng shui, the art and science of placement. Our environment influences our thoughts and our actions, and your biology can either support your life force or drain it.

You've heard of sick buildings where people get headaches or feel depressed and school environments that make it difficult for children to concentrate or learn. In our homes we can have objects that we keep because there is an obligation to another person, and there is a story there of why you keep it. Maybe it belonged to some relative who cherished it, and now you are honoring that person by keeping it. These objects have to be managed energetically and can add stress to your life.

Design and function are not only applicable to work. Have your home set up to be a nurturing environment to support your health and wellness. For example, the living room is a place that we share with others. We can invite friends over and use it as the area for entertainment. When the seats form a U shape and there is a low table, it evokes a kind of campfire feel, where you gather and share in ideas or food. The living room serves a communal function.

Feng shui is an easy way to create harmony and balance with your spouse or partner. In the bedroom, it can create a place for balance and harmony. This is because you share the bed and spend a third of your time sleeping next to each other, and while you are dreaming, your unconscious is vulnerable. It is important that the space be clear of things that don't belong, like exercise machines, computers, piles of clothes, and boxes. Balance is made by making sure you have a table on each side of the bed or reading lamps on each side. A quick harmony fix is to have matching pillowcases.

If there are areas that seem to accumulate "stuff,' there is most likely an energy block. Other objects such as pictures of friends and family probably need to find another place. These create a presence of other people in the room and can subtly disrupt intimacy.

Applying feng shui is an intuitive process and you don't need to take a course in order to start making changes. You can start by clearing out negative energies that do not support your life force (qi), which can very quickly help shift behavioral patterns and thoughts that do not serve you, as well as help create a better space for what it is that you want to focus on, making a difference with fertility. Feng shui is a branch of Chinese medicine, and the principles are about creating your environment to be in harmony with the universal energy and in alignment with your purpose. An example would be if you visit your parents' home and your old room is there, still holding your trophies, posters on the wall, stuffed animals, and princess bedspread. That room is no longer a representation of who you are now; that environment is more of who you were.

One of my patients, Maria, told me how she did not like her apartment; it was her husband's first apartment out of college. The rent was affordable; however, it was more of a bachelor-style living space. There was barely any kitchen area, the living room was long and narrow, you had to go through the bedroom to get to the bathroom, and there was only one closet at the entrance.

She said she did not like to spend time in the apartment, so I asked her to draw me the layout of her apartment and saw that there were some issues with energy flow. However, the biggest issue was in the bedroom, where there was a large, dark wood dresser. The corner of the dresser was pointing at the bed. If you extended the corner, it was like a knife cutting them in two! It was a piece of furniture that needed to go, and not only that, but it had also been in the apartment and left by the previous tenant. The other problem with the big, dark, heavy dresser was that it blocked movement in the room, creating a feeling of being trapped; there would be no space for a baby. Once they got rid of the dresser, the entire apartment felt spacious and light.

HOLDING BOUNDARIES

You have heard about being in the right place at the right time. Well, this is something that applies to your internal and external space.

You can also cleanse people, places, and things. As I mentioned before, pictures of people in the bedroom can feel like an intrusion, so remove them. When you are trying to get pregnant, it is no one's business except for yours and your partner's. When other people get involved, it damages your relationship with yourself and partner, and you will end up feeling pulled in different directions.

Similar to feng shui, the Urban Dictionary definition for "friend shui" is "the art or practice of clearing your life of any friends who cause extra clutter or drama in order to keep a simple, easy, carefree, uplifting social life for yourself." Getting pregnant and having a baby is a big deal, and if there are people in your life who criticize or offer "advice," even if they mean well, that can be a source of stress.

Many people try to be helpful, but they only make matters worse. They might make a comment about adoption or that it's too bad you waited so long or that "Margie got pregnant and she wasn't even trying," and so on. These people don't realize that what they are doing is hurtful, so it is up to you to set the boundaries.

How do you know who to cut out of your fertility journey? Anyone who "makes" you feel bad after an exchange is a person you should cut out. You can't always cut certain people out of your life, but you need to have a plan for when they start giving you advice, especially when it is not asked for. It often comes from out of nowhere; a comment that will catch you off guard and trigger you, and get you reeling for hours or days. Family dynamics can also be a place of passive aggressive behavior where people do and say things that are hurtful, but you have a choice to not participate in gatherings or to limit the time you spend in them.

Create a list of those incidences in the past and identify what was said and how you felt about it. It is important to look at what the trigger was, because that is a clue to where you will work on your fertility mind-set. Next, write out a response to that situation. For example, if there was a comment about "Margie" getting pregnant without trying, imagine you are back in that situation and write out a response to that comment. Also write out a statement that you will say to people who start to pry. As an example, you could write, "I know you mean well, but this is not a conversation I will continue with you," or, "As soon as I have information on this topic, you will be the first to know."

You decide what you want to share, so limit the talk about having a baby and only share what you are doing with a select few. Create your own advisor board with experts who will support your journey, but first you have to be clear about the negative energies that block you so you can remove them.

A woman I worked with used to share with her mother every week what was going on with her and how she and her husband wanted to have a baby, but when she would get off the phone, she felt *bad*. She couldn't figure out why speaking with her mother, which should have been a place of comfort, was in fact making her feel worse! She said, "I feel like shit after talking to my mother. I want to vomit. I can't understand what that was about." It wasn't until she was able to recognize that the relationship she had with her mother was one based on shared misery, talking about how terrible a work situation was, that she realized it created a negative dynamic of victimhood and how the world was against them. There were many old patterns of worthiness and unhealthy dynamics that were always there, but they emerged and came into the light when she started on her journey to becoming a mother. Once she realized what was happening, she had to keep her conversations short and light. She would end the conversations as soon as she would start to feel bad.

I use this example because, in many cases, you don't have to know what they said, but know that it is somehow creating a negative energy and interferes with hope and optimism, which are part of a fertility mind-set. My client identified some self-talk that would show up, seeming like a logical suggestion. Here is a hint: much of your negative thought patterns come from upbringing and experiences.

FERTILITY MIND-SET EXERCISE

Your fertility is not the business of your in-laws, your parents, the teachers you work with, your cousins, your siblings, the yoga studio, the supermarket clerk, or the next-door neighbor. Will they be talking about you, speculating, or judging? *Absolutely*. This is where you will decide your boundaries and that is what we do to create the fertility mind-set. Shifting to a fertility mind-set means becoming aware of where the negative talk is and removing and replacing it with what you want.

You also have to be aware of the circumstances that are also triggers. For instance, if you tell yourself, "I'm too old," you need to replace that thought with something like, "my body is healthy and strong."

Get out of the "chat rooms"; they are filled with other people's fears, and as discussed earlier, we look to "like" others and can take on other people's fears and problems. This is because we have the ability to share another's perspective and experience what they experience; that is how our mirror neurons work to involve empathy. In this case, we have to be careful that we don't step so far into someone else's struggle that it becomes our own. While groups can be helpful, they can also be places of despair and hostility. As you live through others' suffering, you can end up taking on other people's fears. This can create even more of a feeling of isolation.

A patient was recovering from an eating disorder, and she would binge and purge, so as part of her healing process, she connected to some support groups. In the group, the participants would share their struggles of how they would hide their behavior from family, friends, and roommates. My patient shared with me that she felt more isolated, more hopeless, and what was even more difficult was that she learned about new ways that she could hide her activities. This is not the case with all chat rooms and support groups, but they are often not helpful and will be a distraction as well as a time suck.

Similarly, it is hard to hear what a doctor says. It is hard to challenge someone in a white coat and stethoscope, and when they say something, it can be devastating. However, remember that there is truth and then there is *your* truth.

Deborah, a patient of mine, had been through numerous IUI and IVF cycles in the state that she and her husband lived, she was forty-one. While visiting New York on a sabbatical with her husband, they decided to do one last round of IVF at a clinic in New York City. A colleague recommended Deborah come work with me to help her relax and to use the power of acupuncture and Chinese medicine to increase her chances of a successful pregnancy that would result in a healthy baby.

She told me how she tried everything and that this would be their last cycle, and if it didn't happen, then that was that. What she also shared with me that was "disturbing" were the conversations with the doctors at the IVF clinic. They told her that her eggs were no good and that she had a low chance of getting pregnant at all and gave a list of all the problems in regard to why she would probably not be able to succeed. The doctor went so far as to tell her that maybe she just wasn't "meant" to bear a child. These conversations haunted and distressed her, as you can imagine.

I told her not to listen to what they were saying! If there is a God, the doctors are not it. Doctors are looking at their patients from their lens of what they believe *they* can do and how *they* will try to solve this "problem." There is truth, but it is not *your truth*.

In response, we need to create a "filter of heal." This is where it is important to develop that fertility mind-set, which is courage and strength in the face of negativity and not letting anyone or anything squash that light of becoming a mother. It will help you focus on what is going to help you get pregnant and stick with it.

So, what happened to Deborah? We worked together, clearing these negative patterns that were inside, and we also worked on aligning her mind/body and biology with acupuncture and the principles of Chinese medicine.

For this last IVF cycle, she produced three eggs and they were beautiful eggs. The doctor even said, "These are beautiful eggs!"

Yes, she did conceive, and she delivered a beautiful, happy, and healthy baby.

In the next chapter, we will cover how easily we can become discouraged by things that have been said to us and hidden beliefs that we have. These become energetic barriers and can drain your energy and focus. They go unnoticed because they have been around you for a long time and don't seem to bother you. Though they seem like no big deal, you want to be able to clear any negative energy that can be blocking you from getting pregnant.

10

NEGATIVE ENERGY BLOCKS

I call this chapter "the can of worms," because when you are trying to get pregnant, and it is not happening according to "plan," the unravelling starts, and the shit can hit the fan.

With most couples, it is the woman who takes the initiative to look into getting pregnant. She will stop taking birth control if she is on it, and just figures if she and her partner have sex without protection, they should get pregnant in a few months.

Here is where the fear of getting pregnant for most of your life has led you to believe that if you have unprotected sex you get pregnant instantly. This is something that girls and boys are taught in middle school so they don't engage in sexual activities because it could end in an unintended pregnancy and bring shame on them and their families. With that being said, the expectation of immediate success and being met with the reality of failure can rock your world. You might start to feel like things are not what they should be and a thought that maybe you waited too long or that something is wrong with you can come to mind.

When getting pregnant doesn't happen, some doubts about and concerns around ovulation and timing may get your attention and lead you to downloading an app in order to track your cycle a little closer while still being casual about it. What I notice is the idea of "trying" conflicts with a romantic notion of how getting pregnant should just happen naturally. By the time an investment in an ovulation monitor happens, many women have realized that getting pregnant may take longer than they expected, and stress and tension starts to build.

If you want to have a baby, then having sex to make a baby is about timing. Knowing when you are most fertile is a measurable process. You can plan a romantic dinner, and it is always better when care is taken to make sure everything goes smoothly. However, when it comes to getting pregnant, the notion of wanting sex to be spontaneous can cause a lot of stress, and that will also create negative energy and hurt feelings. It is a kind of madness that sets in – overwhelming feelings, crying, screaming, sleepless nights, senseless arguments, and obsessive thoughts. After a while trying to conceive can become extremely nerve-racking and bring out the ugly parts of ourselves.

When women come to see me, they are at the point where they have tried to conceive au naturel and it hasn't happened. Often, they are doing everything in their power to get pregnant. They stop drinking coffee, they stop drinking alcohol, they change their diets, they take supplements, and they may even get their spouse to take some vitamins as well, but something else is going on. So I have to ask them, "Are you leading the charge?"

ARE YOU LEADING THE CHARGE?

There is no reason why you can't schedule a romantic evening around your most fertile time, it's just that worry and anxiety over getting pregnant can take over. In fact, that is why I suggest turning it into a special event, not a chore.

No matter how strong a relationship is, couples who struggle with infertility will feel strain. Husbands and spouses can feel helpless and isolated because they just don't know what to do to make it better.

If you've ever seen a bridezilla, something overtakes these women as they plan out their weddings, and when something does not go according to plan, they turn into bridezilla. This phenomenon has also become a reality show, and so the sensationalism is over the top with women on the verge of a nervous breakdown over a wedding. The point of this is that when you want something badly, it can create a form of temporary insanity, where everything is dramatic because the frustration of not getting pregnant and moving on to the next phase of your life is blocked, and you can't figure out what is blocking you. This is placing conditions on *how* you want it to happen, and those expectations can conflict with what you need to focus on

You may also feel like you are not getting the support that you need or that no one understands what you are going through, or maybe you believe that your partner should read your mind and understand that you are suffering. You might think the doctors you go to see are cold and callous with their statics, and they tap into the deep fear that maybe you cannot get pregnant and have a child and that this might even ruin your marriage or partnership. You might also think something you have wanted your whole life is being taken from you. This is called "secret suffering." I call this secret suffering because you may not even realize that you are suffering. *Fear* is ever present in the background of this insanity, and it usually runs into a deep belief about what it will mean if you cannot get pregnant and have a baby. Will your husband leave you? Will you be deemed broken? Perhaps you would not have been a good parent. Does it mean that you don't deserve to have a baby? As much as you want to have a baby, there are negative energy blocks that show up and have little to do with the biology other than it is being influenced.

As much as you may want to become a mother, this is an unknown, and where there is unknown territory, fear shows up as anxiety and stress – fear about being a good mom, a parent, a wife, a daughter, a teacher, an aunt, a niece, and so on. Yes, all that shit.

If any of these thoughts give you a feeling of dread, to explore them. Write them out in the form of a question. Am I afraid of (fill in the blank)? Do I believe (fill in the blank)?

Seeing a fear on paper takes away the power that you have allowed it to have over you and can now name what it is. Here is where there may be some deeper work to be done to overcome some of your hidden beliefs and fears that undermine your progress.

You are looking to transform a part of yourself, and that will change your whole being and change all of your relationships. Once you have a baby, life does not go back. A butterfly cannot go back to being a caterpillar.

HIDDEN BELIEFS

A big energy block with getting pregnant is not as much with your partner as much as it is with your parents. The relationships you have with yourself and family and what it means can be a can of worms. There are often some energy strings that are still attached to being a certain way, such as wanting to please them, to be perfect, and avoid having shame and guilt. Unresolved issues about being a mother just *stop* everything and make you feel stuck.

Do you have the support you need for getting pregnant? It may mean that you have to sit down with your partner or husband and find out if you are on the same page. From both sides, I have witnessed couples in which the male feels paralyzed and doesn't know what to do to help his wife as she is consumed by the quest of getting pregnant. I have also witnessed husbands who start to become distant and numb to the process and check out because they feel that nothing they do is right. Women tend to be the focus of infertility problems, but 40 percent of infertility problems are related to male infertility.

Marie and her husband, Mike, had separate bank accounts and then a shared account for home, mortgage, utilities, and car payments – basically everything that they shared. However, with regard to fertility, it was completely her expense. This also meant that Marie and her husband didn't have clear communication about what they were going to do with regard to proceeding with fertility treatments. They seemed to be in agreement with spending if it was for a new car that she wanted or to treat her family, but the area of investing in fertility had not been discussed in any detail. With most couples, they may plan for retirement, have a slush fund, or have an emergency fund, but they have not thought about setting money aside for fertility. Money is a vehicle of power, carrying a lot of symbolic and energetic power. Financial commitment – even a small portion – makes a difference. Otherwise, it further creates the idea that getting pregnant is the woman's responsibility and hers alone.

It is crucial that you and your partner are on the same page; otherwise this is a negative energy block that will create a lot of stress and can lead to blame all around. Sometimes women expect the man to just know or be a mind reader, but often he doesn't know how to emotionally support his spouse. Men have been taught a set of rules about "women's issues" and will not necessarily approach the subject unless women invite them in and share. Marie had feelings of shame with her body, and that made it difficult to talk about the depth of her suffering when she wasn't getting pregnant. These feeling made her want to hide and avoid the topic she needed to talk about with her husband. Marie wanted her husband to show her that he supported her and the choices she would make regarding fertility because he understood how important it was for her to become a mom and for Mike to become a father.

Marie got the courage to have a conversation about their future and what was on the vision board for both of them. The energy around who pays for what shifted, as having a baby was a shared goal and became a priority. As a result, they could work out finances.

The health and wellness of both people in a committed relationship impact their bond. It needs to be looked at as a shared investment for the future of their happiness. With regard to your partner, what should he be doing instead? What do you want instead?

We can often have a narrative or story about our partner that they don't want to help or care. It comes from a place of being a victim as a woman. We take on the burdens and the cultural stereotypes and don't leave an opening for our partner to participate. I recommend that both of you work on a vision board of what you both desire and include the baby. Do it on Pinterest, so you can share it with each other. Include everything, house, car, vacation, and symbols of what is important.

Get support from your work as well. Do you have the type of career or occupation that you have time for yourself? If you are in a job that makes demands of your time, trying to get pregnant or thinking about how you will have a baby becomes another barrier.

In the previous chapter, we talked about creating boundaries and priorities, and work tends to be a source of difficulty. If you have been trying to keep appointments with a fertility clinic early in the morning and your job requires you to travel or your partner to travel, it will definitely make getting pregnant more challenging. This kind of situation can cause you to develop resentment and feel like the world is against you.

At the same time, there is a lot of insanity that gets infused into some of this process. This may not be happening to you, but it can feel like you are the only one that is doing everything right and no one else is on board, which can also create tremendous stress. In the previous chapter where I asked you to write out your to do list, if you are in a place where you do everything yourself, take a pause and make sure that on your priority list your relationship with your spouse or partner is being nurtured. If you already know that both of you have stressful jobs and commitments, the exercise for priority and urgency needs to be done again with your partner.

ANGER AND RESENTMENT

I hate to imply that men don't care, but they have a different biology, and they never have the same pressure that they are getting old and should start having kids. Therein can be why you feel like it could be the end of the world if your spouse may seem distant and possibly unsympathetic.

Anger and resentment are major energy blocks that are very destructive. The pressure of getting pregnant builds, and everywhere you turn it can seem like everyone else is having success except for you. When that happens, the fertility madness takes over and is all-consuming. In some cases, this can destroy a marriage.

When Penny came to see me to help her get pregnant, she was thirty-eight and single. Modern reproductive medicine makes it possible for women that want to become moms to do so, and it makes it possible for same sex couples to become parents regardless of gender. She had done several rounds of IUIs that had not been successful, so she decided to take a break from the hormones and figure out when to go back to try another cycle or change clinics altogether. I admired Penny's courage and that she was calm about the process.

Penny had been married for five years, and she and her husband had tried to get pregnant for the last two years of their marriage, but with each cycle failing and then doing fertility cycles at a clinic, their relationship had started to fracture. There had been a lot of fighting about things like what was for dinner, that in the big picture were not important and had become blown out of proportion. Their marriage and life had started to revolve around doctor appointments and ovulation. Vacations could not be planned because it might conflict with one of the cycles. They had stopped having sex for intimacy and connection because it was all about making a baby and working around a clinic schedule. After each argument, they never really recovered, so resentment built up and being together in the same room what cause tension. It was right before they were scheduled to do an IVF that her husband said he had enough and wasn't going to go through with it. He said he never really cared about having a child. This was a devastating blow. They filed for divorce, and she never saw or heard from him again.

What was left was a lot of anger and resentment toward her ex-husband. She felt that if she had known that he never wanted children, maybe she wouldn't have married him or she would have separated from him sooner because not wanting a child was a deal breaker. Now she was doing the process on her own. Nothing would stop her because she wanted a baby. The problem was that there was anger and resentment and residual negative energy that would bubble up and envelop her. Her throat would tighten, and she felt pain in her chest and was experiencing constipation. She could not forgive what happened and it was blocking her. She could sense this as well.

We are very powerful beings and our emotions are energy. Energy moves matter and accumulates, unless you release it. Physically some tiny fibroids had started to grow, and with fertility hormones they can get bigger. Penny was aware that these negative thought forms had power and that she needed to release them because every time she thought of her past it kept her in that negative energy. Her throat, heart, and uterus energy centers were blocked.

The work we did together was to open the flow of qi and blood and to release the emotions that were trapped. We also had her remove her husband's name from her phone and contact list and cut ties with people that report back on what her ex-husband is doing. Taking those actions helped her release negative energy and make space for love that she could give to a baby.

You hold within you a lot of power and energy; it can be influenced by your environment, people, objects, and your past experience. In the next chapter, we will be exploring how elements of feng shui, the art and science of placement, affect your life force and what you can do to create a nurturing and healing environment to support your relationship and fertility.

11

CREATION AND FERTILITY FENG SHUI

When I talk to my patients about using feng shui to help with fertility and how feng shui has cures, they definitely lean in. There is a lot of mystery around the practice of feng shui. What I can tell you is that it is a branch of Chinese medicine, and just as the use of acupuncture helps move the energy blockages that are in meridians in your body to create the free flow of qi, feng shui plays a key role in fertility as well.

We are energetic bodies and we have physical, energetic, emotional, and spiritual aspects to us; technically, we are all of these things at the same time. Just as in quantum physics, we are many things at once; therefore, we are a part of everything at the same time.

How can you use feng shui? This is an exercise in creation; what you can imagine or desire comes first and then can come to fruition when you take action and start to make the thing in a representational form.

Having a baby is something that is creation, and setting your environment up for that to be successful is what you can do. First, what will this look like? Your dream of having that baby is maybe all jumbled with thoughts of what you want. At the same time, you have pictures and thoughts of why you can't have it, like age or believing you are broken. That will make it difficult to have the strong "knowing," the energy of staying on course in the face of disappointments or other people's fears and ideas. You want to be absolutely clear about what you want and no one else can take that desire from you. This is an ongoing theme that we have covered in previous chapters, and it always needs to be a reminder. I am repeating this because often the same thoughts and doubts come up again and again as we move through different steps. These negative thoughts are painful because they are the ones that we continue to tell ourselves. The fertility mindset is a continuous exercise and is there to help you when you feel doubt or resistance.

Just as the architect draws the design and builds the model, you have to create what you want in a representation. First, you want to get a feeling of certainty. Just as you are certain that the sun will rise tomorrow, you want to have that feeling. You may not have ever realized how things come to fruition; they sometimes seem like luck. However, luck is opportunity meeting preparedness, and I look at everything that we do as preparation for what we want. The thing is that no one ever tells you that there is a secret to all this. People have gone from poverty to riches with an idea that got built in a garage and later became a laptop and smartphone sitting in your hands. Someone had a vision and an idea of what they wanted and had to hold that vision and determination to move forward and toward it.

If you have ever done sewing, knitting, baking, home designing, or wedding planning, the example here is that you have an image – an idea of what you want to have – and with the materials you have, you make that come together to become a "creation." With this same feel of "knowing," you connect to something greater, and then you proceed to the next task.

There was an exercise from a previous chapter to first create a Pinterest board with everything – your partner, house, car, vacations, preschools – you envision with having this baby. Make it as creative as possible; don't judge the process. This is a vision board, and you must include everything from holidays to christenings, with all the bells and whistles. If you did not do it before or thought it was silly, it is not; you can create a new one or look at the one you made and make some edits.

I recommend that you make a new vision board and take some of those elements that you still like to help you to get into that *feeling* of certainty, the feeling you felt when you knew that you were in love or that made you decide you wanted a particular career or to live in a particular city. Additionally, use a picture of a baby. I recommend finding a picture that makes your heart ache, like the feeling you get when you see little puppies or cute animals that make you want to pick them up or have one. It is that clear feeling of desire and love, something that you want to love. These strong feelings can conjure every time you look at the photo. They make you feel that it "is" your baby.

You will also want to use feng shui in your bedroom. Why is this so important? You spend at least six to seven hours there a night while you sleep and can use that as a focus point and energy concentration. My suggestion is that you do a layout sketch and look at where everything is. People tend to have a lot of stuff in their bedroom. It may seem unimportant because you spend time in your bedroom sleeping, but this is a big mistake, and it can disrupt your relationship and energetically block you from getting pregnant.

Clear any clutter that is in your bedroom, especially if there is an exercise machine, TV screen, or computer there as these are big distractions. One of the tenants of feng shui is that energy flows and will support you. Computers and TV screens give off electromagnetic frequency, and studies show that these radioactive frequencies affect sleep hormones and reproductive hormones like luteinizing (ovulation) and also are linked to cellular breakdown.

The other thing about screens is that they are a two-way window, making you feel that the whole world is in your bedroom, so you are not alone. In a weird way, it is like there is another presence or a ghost. If you cannot move it, then cover it so it is not "looking" at you.

Remove mirrors that reflect you as you sleep because mirrors reflect energy, and if you are worried, or having restless sleep, it will intensify the energy. If there is clutter or disarray, it will also magnify that energy. You want to have your bedroom serve as a sanctuary away from all of the stressors and reminders of tasks that have to do with work or other people.

Get rid of clutter under your bed, as this creates stagnation and can represent "stuff" you don't want to deal with but is still there. It can be challenging if you don't have a lot of storage space but clearing under the bed is kind of like getting rid of the skeletons in the closet.

If you have objects that remind you that you need to do something else, these will scatter your energy and create stress; remove those as well. When entering the bedroom, the energy should slow down a bit and allow you to feel calm and settled.

On either side of the bed, you want to have a table or nightstand and a light. They should be in pairs, and they do not have to match, but the reason they are in pairs is for balance and harmony. Visually it is pleasing, but really this balance is about male and female energy. The balance of yin and yang is about the energy of light and dark and nature's cycle.

In addition, the light in your bedroom should be soft and low, as this will signal your brain to make melatonin, known as the dark hormone, that signals your body to start to relax and rest. Getting into a calm state is how we are able to go from being stressed out to a state of rest and digest, supporting the reproductive cycle. Studies show the effect of light on ovulation in the morning, signaling alignment with the natural cycle of the day. As we head into the evening, we need dimmer light so that the sleep cycle is not interrupted.

While the bed should face the direction of the door, it should not be directly in front of the door, so if you are lying in bed, you will see if someone enters. This means you are not taken by surprise and energy entering the doorway will slow down. If the bed is in front of the door, you will feel like something is speeding into the room, and there is no privacy. If needed, you can use the Japanese split curtains that are placed in doorways so when they are open, they still provide a little screen.

The colors of the room should be calming and more on the neutral side, reflecting what you would like to feel. If you want the room to feel warm, go with earth tones; if you want a healing energy, add more blues or greens.

Put art and pictures on the walls, choosing art to reflect what you want to feel. With pictures, keep only ones of you and your partner. If you have photos of other people, as I mentioned before, it is like having them in the room with you, and I don't recommend it; you can place them in another room.

If you are wondering whether any of this feng shui stuff works or not, I can tell you that it definitely does. All cultures engage in a form of the art of living, and in Asian culture, feng shui has been implemented for over five thousand years with the understanding of the energies of the universe and how they play out in our environment in and outside of our homes, offices, markets, streets, and cities. There are more and more studies linking how space organization and design can positively impact productivity, mental health, and our well-being.

For young children, a well-designed classroom will facilitate learning and better behavior because it takes into account what the needs are, and the space facilitates the activities. Modern-day city planners can look at traffic patterns and look to ease them by changing directions or creating traffic circles to keep a city moving.

In terms of fertility, this is generally the same idea, but with the understanding that feng shui can help you be prosperous and promote health and general wellness. If city planners in our Western metropolis implemented these principles, perhaps some of the things that stress us the moment we go out into the world could be alleviated.

THE FENG SHUI CURE

Early on while I was in graduate school, over thirty-five, and also in the process of trying to conceive, I had the good fortune of meeting a feng shui master who was also a Chinese medicine practitioner in the true sense. Learning from him was an enlightening experience. Everything he taught had clarity, like clouds parting and the sun shining through with rainbows. I asked him about having a baby, and he looked at me and said that I needed a feng shui cure, and this is what I did, and I also share with my patients.

Take that picture of the baby, the one that makes your heart ache, and one picture of you and one of your partner and put the picture of the baby in between the photos, wrap a red ribbon around it, and place it under your mattress. What this does is tells the universe that the desire is clearly here. The mother and father together, just waiting for the baby. The fact that you are in one place for six to seven hours helps to manifest what you desire. Of course, you have to do your part, such as having relations during your fertile time.

This feng shui cure needs to be done with conviction. If you don't get into the energy or do the activity, then do not do it. It is something that is there to help you hold that energy.

One of my clients, Eloise, exclaimed, "I had completely forgotten that it was there until it flew out when we flipped the mattress!" The photo was placed under the mattress while she was getting acupuncture to help regulate her cycle after a miscarriage and IVF.

Eloise and her husband had been trying to have a baby for some time. They were both business professionals, and with each passing month, there was mounting worry and fear. Having a placeholder for their wishes of becoming parents helped both of them stay optimistic about their chances of getting pregnant.

She and her husband did get pregnant and have a healthy baby boy.

When she told me that she had found the photo, it was a surprise to her, because she had done the exercise and forgot about it. I believe that the message to the universe was received.

I worked with another couple on the West Coast, and both husband and wife were on their second marriages. Lily was thirty-nine and Jim was forty-eight. Lily was ambivalent about having children, but after three years, she changed her mind, and they did not want to go the route of IVF or IUI, so they embarked on getting healthy and doing whatever they could to improve their fertility. The great part was that Jim was 110 percent committed and on board with doing all the exercises of the vision boards and the feng shui cure.

We decided to try implementing an additional feng shui cure by creating an altar. Creating an altar is another way to call in energy, and it is something that if you want to do it, you can. If you come from a Christian background, this may feel uncomfortable like you are practicing voodoo or witchcraft. Do the exercises that resonate with your beliefs. What we say to ourselves every day is praying to God or the Universe, which is why your thoughts, words, and deeds need to be in alignment.

Together, they chose a picture of a baby they both felt drawn to, and a part of the exercise was to place an offering to the baby. It could be a pair of booties, a pacifier, or a baby blanket. This was to "call in" that they were ready to receive and take care of a child, and this was to be done every day along with a little prayer in four directions North, South, East and West. The four directions call on the energy of the elements Earth, Fire, Air and Water to come together. Lo and behold, they became pregnant with twins when Lily was forty-two, and she delivered right before she turned forty-three. Jim shared with me that every day, he said the prayers. When the twins were born, he sent a picture of the altar they had created, and that was when I noticed that he had placed two silver rattles on the altar!

I want to emphasize how powerful working with feng shui can be, especially when a couple is unified, and they work together with intention and creation energies. The results are miraculous.

In the next chapter, I give more details of how the energies of the universe are working and ways for you to use them to get pregnant.

12

THE WAY OF HEAVEN

The Way of Heaven describes a state of being physically, energetically, emotionally, and spiritually in alignment. You may have called it another name like being in the flow or synchronicity, and I know that everyone has had this feeling where everything just comes together and works "perfectly." Getting pregnant are those energies of desire, the openness of the heart and mind, and the physical readiness to receive and allow for the miracle of life to come through you.

In all cultures, there are many beliefs about fertility and health. Many spiritual texts are guides for living a healthy life in body, mind, and spirit. Living in a science-dominated culture, many of these ideas are considered woo woo and not taken seriously. After all, they do resemble witchcraft and we have been taught that it is evil or to be suspicious of power that cannot be explained.

Luckily the law of attraction and The Secret has gain awareness in the mainstream and helps to bring the ideas of on universal principles of alignment with consciousness and action.

WHAT I HAVE FOUND IS THAT WHEN WOMEN AND COUPLES TRY to conceive, they go so far into science that they become separated from the energy of creation. The focus is so much on physical health, what's not working, and what must be wrong, that it disconnects the line to the universe and the energy of life, qi.

What you need to understand about the universe is that the baby you want is already here. The same molecules that make up the chair you sit on and the table you write on are the same that makes up a plant, metal, water, and, yes, a human. You were already born with the eggs you have. In fact, they were percolating in your mom when she was in your grandmother's womb! Your spouse or partner has the sperm; all the ingredients are here. The big question is, What is it that directs those molecules to come together in a particular way to then use the materials from your body and convert them into a human being?

Some scientific statistics say that the chance of you being born as you are 1 in 400 trillion. I think the odds of winning a lottery ticket are better, yet here you are.

While life appears to be chaotic, there has to be a matrix of balance that we are a part of. This is where the Daoist principles come from, the balance of *yin* and *yang*. We tend to think in black and white, either or, but yin and yang are a dynamic balance, and when we talk about making a baby, that is exactly what happens. A little bit of each of the two of you mixed together in just the right measure and at just the right time – not necessarily the time you want, but the time that is right.

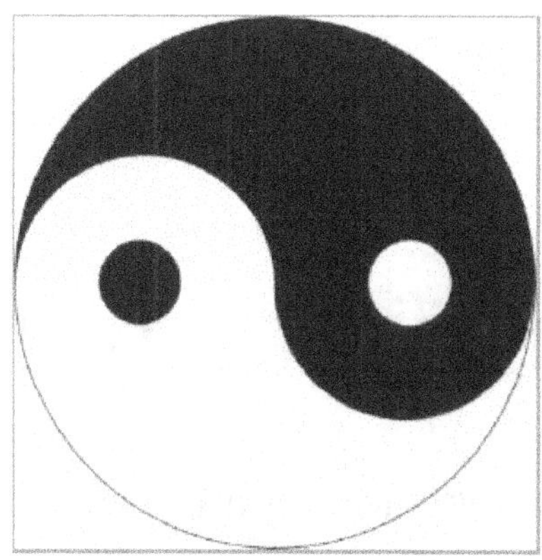

The Daos believed optimal health (fertility) could be attained by practicing the Dao, also known as the "way." They understood the principles of practicing the "way" as balancing the transformation of the energies of the universe through physical, energetic, emotional, and spiritual levels.

As esoteric as this may sound, what I have come to understand is that the meaning is literal. What the Daoist means is this is about the universe within you. When you align with your physical, energetic, and emotional aspects, you can open yourself to the spiritual energies or the universal matrix. This is a clear path to be able to receive the energy that tells those molecules to create a life. It involves being in the right place at the right time; you might call this "luck," or opportunity meets preparedness.

Connecting your energy with your partner means both of you are in sync, not just eggs and sperm, but with the preconceived vision of what you are creating. This is an energy of knowing and being and not the frantic energy of "trying and trying."

How will that work? In the previous chapter, we covered some of the obstacles that show up in a relationship when the focus on trying to have a baby hijacks and causes isolation in relationships. Including your partner in creating a vision board and sharing the journey helps to create a deep connection helps to remind you of the reason that you are together.

An exercise to help join your energies.

BREATHING TECHNIQUE

After practicing a breathing technique, one of my patients told me, "My husband was a bit resistant to doing the breathing technique; he thought it was silly when I talked about it, and felt a bit awkward, but I wanted to try. He agreed he would do it for me. At first, it took some time to feel comfortable, and I was worried about doing it the right way, but then I just started breathing. If I got a little squirmy, I was worried he would give up, so I relaxed into it. When we opened our eyes and looked at each other, it was such a strange feeling; I felt like I was seeing him for the first time. I noticed the angle of his jaw, the direction his hair was flowing and the gentle wave it had, the little creases on the side of his eyes, and his long lashes as he smiled, though trying to be serious. I could see what he looked like as a little boy, so sweet, and the thought that our baby would have his soft brown eyes. I could see it and feel it now."

I will share with you this same breathing technique. This is a simple exercise for couples to do before going to bed, not necessarily before sex, but to synchronize energy. Sit across from each other on the floor or bed, cross legged, eyes closed, and holding hands, begin breathing slowly, inhaling through the nose and exhaling out the mouth. Try breathing at the same rate and rhythm. This can take two to three minutes, and you will notice the energy flowing in your body. You can then open your eyes and gently gaze into each other's eyes. You might feel a bit self-conscious or silly but do it anyway. Notice all the features on your partner's face and continue to breathe together. You may begin to feel energy and pulsing in your hands and you can imagine energy flowing from your right arm through your hand to your partner and your left-hand receiving energy from your partner. Feel it flow through both your bodies. It is a powerful feeling and you can focus on the warmth in your chest (heart center). Let that energy flow down through your body to your lower abdomen and let it flow out toward you partner, having him also imagine this. As you are breathing in and out, every one of your seventy trillion cells are oxygenating until all your cells are breathing at the same time.

This exercise is practicing the energy of love from your heart center and connects it with your creative center in the womb. In Chinese medicine, this is called the *Bao Mai*, the extra pathway of the heart and uterus. Some couples can feel their bodies expand and connect to everything; they are becoming "one" with the universe.

Why is this exercise important to do? As humans, we go to resonate with other people's vibrations. If others are strong and calm, we tend to get relaxed and feel safe. We go to match others; that is why, when we are in a crowd and everyone is excited, we feel excited, just as much as we can feel panic or fear go around. Your vibration is a big part of the creative energy and fertility.

There is also an aspect of detachment from the outcome. As much as you want it to happen, there is surrender to the process and energy of receiving, not the energy of getting.

Doing this exercise every evening for ten to fifteen minutes is excellent for destressing and clearing your mind of the monkey chatter and clutter, and you will sleep better. When you do the exercise together, you support each other in a kind of meditation. Each of you sets the pace and that makes it easier to follow. It is also a segue from electronics to a state of relaxation. You and your partner will be attuned to each other's energy, and when you are at your most fertile time, the tension around getting pregnant will be released.

THE FERTILITY RITUAL

You have heard about couples who were trying for years and gave up to later get pregnant by accident or without even trying. I don't believe it is completely true that it was an accident; there had to be that moment where they connected with each other that opened the door for the spiritual and creative energy to be allowed in. Because trying to conceive tends to create more stress and take the romance out of sex, it becomes a chore. Instead, create a ritual.

Doing this exercise and then creating a fertility ritual during your fertile time marks a celebration. Clear your calendars and eat the foods you love, use scented candles or essential oils, take a ritual bath, and make it something you both look forward to. You are invoking something divine, and it is important to make it special and divine.

By practicing connecting with yourself and your partner, the energies of the universe or the way of heaven, form as one in mind, body, and spirit in the creative process of life. The molecules of life become drawn to the place that they can form.

Yin and yang are dynamic balance that you influence with everything that you do whether conscious of it or not. Breathing and connecting in a ritual with your partner is a conscious action that results in creation that is not random.

What I have shared in this chapter is a way to work with creative energy and the energy of life to create the conditions that will help you get pregnant. Success with using the steps that I have shared with you will help you if you do them and do not give into to doubt or old patterns. In the next chapter, I will go cover what might stop you from continuing or doing these exercises.

13

THE GREAT LEAP FORWARD

Moving from being in a place of failure and feeling stuck to alignment and enlightened action is a great leap forward. The steps to take are simple and doable; that is the beauty of the process. Where people fail is when they approach their problem the same way, and they don't even realize it. No matter how badly you want to have a baby, there are circumstances and things that can get in your way of success. The frustrating part is that you don't know they are there and they always seem to have a "good reason." These are invisible forces that seem like they make sense and are not the problem but looking at where they show up and how they can get you to stop yourself is important.

What can happen is something called "magic bullet syndrome;" it shows up to get you to stop. This is where there you have the belief that having a baby occurs by a mysterious force that is conjured by doing some of the steps conception, and then magically, this brings you results.

The simplest and smallest shifts take time to implement and for your body, mind, and spirit to synchronize to where you get it and it becomes easy. Studies show that it is a minimum of twenty-one days and up to almost a year to get into a rhythm. This has to do with setting your neurology up and implementing time-spaced repetition. Time spaced repetition is how we learn new habits and create grooves in our brain. Think of playing a musical instrument or learning a new language, or a little baby that learns to crawl. These things take thousands and thousands of repetition before successful coordination occurs. If you feel like you don't have enough time, this will be a place to look at what might make you give up.

If it feels like hard work, resistance, and doubt set in, and you can lose momentum and stop. Make a commitment to have an open mind and don't question your decisions or look for a scientific explanation for why something should or should not work. This gets back into a loop of where you started out and doubt creeps in and you end up giving up.

You need to maintain consistency; this comes from the commitment to keeping positive and open-minded, allowing yourself to make mistakes. When you do the exercises, you create momentum and success that will continue to motivate you. We are rewriting old patterns and they have been around for a long time. Without commitment, doubt slips in if you let it and you can find yourself stopping for no reason, saying, "I don't know. One day, I just stopped."

Another obstacle to success is not prioritizing your fertility and allowing other things to take over. This journey needs to be the priority, and that is done through the commitment you make to yourself to make it a priority. It's like going on a diet and not eating sugar; someone may put cake in front of you and tempt you. Letting other people or things get in the way tells your subconscious that your desire has conditions, and it is not so important. In this way, you don't give it your all. If you say yes to everyone or are a people pleaser, this can leak into putting other people's needs first. If you find you are overscheduled and unwilling to let some of those things go, you will not have enough energy to continue.

For there to be accountability to stay the course with commitment, good planning has to come with it. Decide to hold yourself accountable by setting up a system, such as your calendar, and look at it to see what you need to put in place. An example could be wanting to practice yoga because it will support your mind-body connection. Signing up for classes, clearing your schedule, and maybe enlisting a friend who will encourage you to keep it up or creating a "challenge" will help you stay the course. Having support is a way to be accountable. Enlist your partner or spouse as a way to connect and support both of you. Wouldn't it be amazing to go to yoga together and create your nurturing environment? Without having accountability, old habits can derail your progress and you can lose excitement and perhaps not give it your all.

Not knowing when you should ask for help when you need it is one of those sneaky habits that shows up all the time. You are smart and should be able to figure it out on your own, but that can keep you overwhelmed and in your head, wondering why you are not getting pregnant or your subconscious comes up with some other explanation. Perhaps you feel shame around whether you are "stupid," should know this stuff, or think that it should be easy, and these feelings can cause you to stop your fertility journey. Perhaps you don't monitor and correct the negative internal dialogue that tells you that maybe there is something wrong, that if you were meant to get pregnant, it would have happened or that maybe you don't deserve to have a baby. This is evil monkey chatter that is disguised as scientific reasoning, but it is a hidden belief that shows up a lot. This is why the fertility mind-set is so important. If you don't invoke the fertility mind-set, it is easy to give up.

When I see the spark of potential for a woman to get pregnant and have a beautiful, healthy, and happy baby, it is incredible. Gradually, she discovers those secrets that have been locked away and out of her awareness, and they come alive. She discovers how to put the pieces together for herself like a puzzle, completing a joyful picture. The answer is in front of her and if she sticks with it, she will take action.

I know that if she can commit to the process that she will become so much closer to getting pregnant and having that happy and healthy baby smiling up at her, but the sad part of this is that success is so close, and at the same time, so far. The patterns that keep us searching for the wrong answers and in a place of indecision makes everything so much more difficult. The gift of doing the work helps to overcome invisible barriers, because as you go through the process, they become clearer. There is much to learn, but it is not impossible, and what you will discover is that you will feel good about what you are doing and the choices you make about what helps you. This is your truth. This is your alignment and you are able to understand and remove those energetic blocks. From experience, I can tell you that if those blocks around having a baby are present, they are also impeding other aspects and diminishing the quality of your life and your dreams.

We are working on something so great, your dream come true, and this will bring incredible joy and meaning to your life. I know you have an inkling of what that is, otherwise, you would not be taking this journey. As I've said in the earlier chapters, awareness is the beginning.

14

CONCLUSION

Together, we've been on the journey of trying to get pregnant. When you are forty, you experience stress beyond belief, and you may not have thought having a baby would take this long. This is especially frustrating, as I know you are a smart lady, and not being able to figure it out makes this failure so heartbreaking, and rightly so. Looking outside of the norm is where you finally start to awaken to the fact that all is not what it seems. Even with that pesky statistic that every white coat and stethoscope quotes you seems to follow you around the internet and into every chat room.

Having revealed that much of what you are told by Western medicine, and in particular, fertility clinics, has not been helpful in guiding you toward your dream of having a baby, they are just offering you the best of what they know. But it is not helping you get what you need and ultimately lead you to having that baby. The personal cost is high. Shame, guilt, and regrets of what could have been may even haunt you.

In this book, I shared a bit about my background and my personal experience in the Western model of medicine and how it shaped what I do and how dedicated I am to helping women. While I did not have the same struggles as other women, I know what it feels like to have a baby and how it expands your heart with more love than you could imagine possible. This beautiful experience is something not to be missed. I know what the gift is and that is why I want to help as many women as I can to pull through their suffering and show them how they can come into alignment, because I know it is possible.

The map is not the territory; it exemplifies how we see the world through our filters and that creates a holographic map telling us where to go and how to live our lives. The map is usually designed by someone else or many other people, beliefs, and social constructs that also make it seem like you have no choice. This is a reality that we can choose to believe or recognize the inconsistencies that cast doubt on what you believed.

Truth is something that eventually is revealed if you keep an open mind, and then you find that you have the power within you. I love the moment of reveal when Dorothy from *The Wizard of Oz* confronts the wizard and finds that there is just a man pulling strings of illusion. Her little dog, Toto, was not fooled by the theatrics and helped a surprised Dorothy see the truth of her situation. The scrappy dog ran to the side of the room and started pulling the green curtains hanging on the wall. "Pay no attention to that man behind the curtain," said the man.

Perhaps there are illusions about what the problem is for getting pregnant that have led you to take steps in the wrong direction. Having an open mind and curiosity that there must be other possibilities helps you see other paths and tools that will help you and are missing and that can now be used.

Being seasoned in having gone through some fertility turmoil, you can lose sight of why you are on this journey to getting pregnant and having a baby. Fertility fatigue creeps in and the bigger picture of what it means to become a mother can feel like it's squished. With every failure, the dream seems to be farther and farther away. Renewing the desire and why this is important helps clear away the doubts that can cause despair. A renewed determination and clarity of mission will make taking the next steps easier, along with the exercise describing why you want to have a baby and the vision board exercise.

We looked at some of the most damaging myths that women are told about their fertility that lead them to believe they have no choice for having a baby. They are led to believe that unless it involves taking hormones and getting invasive medical procedures, they will not have a baby. We are looking at a medical system that still treats women as if they are weak and suffering from hysteria. This idea of hysteria is so embedded in our culture that we cannot distinguish it from reality and accept it as a flaw and a curse. Women feel emotional ups and downs, as if they are to blame for not getting pregnant, leading them to more suffering. They feel they are broken and because infertility always starts with looking at a woman's age and uterus, it further perpetuates those myths. Unlearning what we learned is important, as we need to know where information comes from and how we may blindly accept it as truth and fact. Questioning where all this "knowledge" comes from will allow you to disseminate what the truth is for yourself.

So many obstacles show up when we want something big. Getting pregnant is no different and developing a strategy and process for success that meets your individual needs must be put in place. This includes people, things, and responsibilities in the form of obstacles that you have in your neatly packaged life. The way we think we need to be and do things is inaccurate, and that is evident because it's not working for you.

Together, we took a good look at your life and what is important so that you can get pregnant and have a baby. This close examination of how we run our lives is often overlooked, because high achiever and successful and productive people tend to be busy and will overextend themselves. Making getting pregnant a priority means logistical adjustments and adjustments to how you will think about your fertility journey.

In this book, there were also specific exercises so you can get clear on what is a priority versus urgency. I also discussed the importance of getting a clear picture of where you are with your overall health and getting up to date with any tests that offer intel on your reproductive cycle. We need to know the big picture so that we can be in alignment with your desire to have a baby and your health. This means we cannot ignore health conditions, but we can look at how they are specific to your health, creating a plan that you can take action on. Realistically looking at how long something might take to improve and what you can do does not depend on where you are in your fertility journey. Knowledge of your body and how it works puts the power of choice about health and healing into your hands. You know how your body feels because it is yours.

We looked at common health issues that are often overlooked, such as chronic inflammation, like yeast infections, and metabolic and endocrine disruptors, including hormonal birth control. Many are not considered an issue but do raise some red flags as health concerns.

We looked at how doing everything perfectly can cause more stress and impede the process of getting pregnant. There is a myth about doing everything perfectly with regard to fertility and getting pregnant. This leads many women down the road of obsessiveness, compulsion, shame, and self-loathing. We discussed the topic of what women think of themselves and their bodies through how we have been acculturated and how that plays into our ideas of perfection. Our value and self-worth are on the chopping block.

We looked at strategies of how to go into alignment with the body's cycle, looking at what is "normal" instead of trying to force the body into conformity with some medical ideal. Exercises in tracking and monitoring the menstrual cycle without the involvement of electronics were a priority.

I gave you an introduction into the fertility mind-set, how to reset your thinking about getting pregnant, how people can be a source of pain, and how certain activities such as hanging out in chat rooms can cause more emotional strain because we fill our thoughts with other people's struggles. We hold beliefs about how we need to be with family and friends and our emotional boundaries are not clear. This is unlearning much of what we learned about who we are.

You are a kind, sensitive, and empathetic person, and it is natural to reach out and feel empathy for others, but there is a point where it does not help you; in fact, it hurts. You may start to recognize people in your circle who make you feel bad about yourself that you've been tolerating. Creating awareness around how you think and what you say to yourself, especially around getting pregnant, is important to reframe. An exercise for creating a fertility mind-set was introduced as a key for helping you stay on track and to become aware when your thoughts are triggered.

We touched on the dynamics that show up with couples who try to have a baby as well as the stress of failure and how it can lead to feelings of loneliness and feeling as if this burden is all on you. Looking at what it is that both you and your spouse want and including your partner or spouse in this journey will bring you closer instead of driving a wedge between you. Fear is a major theme with infertility, and it is a motivator and destroyer.

If you are leading the charge with fertility, the stress and responsibility will become toxic. We addressed the topic of removing obstacles and going a little deeper into the weeds, looking at the more intimate struggles that may need to be addressed and can take time. If the fertility journey has strained your relationship, that will need some repair and work commitments may need to be reexamined or changed. Areas of our lives tend to get overlooked when the focus is so narrow, such as on fertility alone.

We also discussed the spiritual aspects of Chinese medicine and ancient practices around feng shui and how it affects your overall health and wellness as well as fertility. There are actual activities to engage in for both you and your partner to shift the energy that has a large impact on health and fertility. Doing these exercises with your partner will help to bring you closer as the environment will begin to support your dream of having a happy and healthy baby. Like the vision board exercise with a partner or spouse, the breathing technique is a unified front.

Lastly, we covered the alignment of energies of mind, body, and spirit and how to create that connection with the universe and all the steps and activities to help bring about that connection in partnership. It is something powerful when you step into alignment with the energies of the universe and have your beautiful and healthy baby smiling up at you.

There many possibilities for you to tap into your creative power that is within you and all around you. This greatness is something that has always been a part of you and is what helps to bring a new life into this world. Use the guidelines and exercises in the book to help you stay in the energy of possibility and positivity. Don't worry about doing everything or doing it perfectly. Know if you desire to have that happy and healthy baby, it is already here.